THE GLOBAL CHALLENGE OF HEALTH CARE RATIONING

STATE OF HEALTH SERIES

Edited by Chris Ham, Director of Health Services Management Centre, University of Birmingham

THE GLOBAL CHALLENGE OF HEALTH CARE RATIONING

EDITED BY
**Angela Coulter and
Chris Ham**

Open University Press
Buckingham · Philadelphia

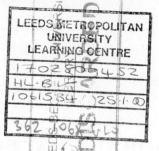
Open University Press
Celtic Court
22 Ballmoor
Buckingham
MK18 1XW

email: enquiries@openup.co.uk
world wide web: http://www.openup.co.uk

and
325 Chestnut Street
Philadelphia, PA 19106, USA

First Published 2000

A catalogue record of this book is available from the British Library

ISBN   0 335 20463 5 (pbk)   0 335 20464 3 (hbk)

Library of Congress Cataloging-in-Publication Data
The global challenge of health care rationing/edited by Angela
Coulter and Chris Ham.
    p. cm.   (State of health series)
  ISBN 0-335-20464-3 (hbk)   ISBN 0-335-20463-5 (pbk)
  1. Health care rationing. 2. Medical economics—Moral and ethical
aspects. 3. Health planning. Moral and ethical aspects. I. Coulter,
Angela. II. Ham, Chris. III. Series.
    RA394.9 .G56 2000
    362.1 dc21   99-32133
                                                                 CIP

Typeset by Type Study, Scarborough
Printed in Great Britain by St Edmundsbury Press, Bury St Edmunds,
Suffolk

CONTENTS

LIST OF CONTRIBUTORS

Vittorio Bertelè is Head of the Regulatory Policies Laboratory at the Istituto di Ricerche Farmacologiche Mario Negri, Milan.

John Bryant is Emeritus Professor in the Department of Community Health Sciences at the Aga Khan University, Karachi, Pakistan and President of the Council of International Organizations for Medical Sciences, Geneva.

David Chinitz is Lecturer in the Department of Medical Management, Economics and Ecology at the Hebrew University Hadassah, School of Public Health, Jerusalem.

Carolyn Clancy is Director of the Center for Outcomes and Effectiveness Research at the Agency for Health Care Policy and Research, Department of Health and Human Services, Rockville MD.

Joanna Coast is Lecturer in Health Economics in the Department of Social Medicine at the University of Bristol, Bristol.

Angela Coulter is Director of Policy and Development at the King's Fund, London.

Norman Daniels is Goldthwaite Professor in the Department of Philosophy at Tufts University, Medford MA.

Marion Danis is Senior Researcher in the Department of Clinical Bioethics at the National Institute of Health, Bethesda MD.

Elizabeth Dennett is Lecturer and Research Fellow at the Department of Surgery, Faculty of Medicine and Health Science at the University of Auckland.

Wendy Edgar is Programme Director of the National Advisory Committee on Health and Disability, Wellington.

Noya Galai is Senior Lecturer in the Department of Epidemiology at Ben Gurion University, Beer Sheva.

Silvio Garattini is Director of the Istituto di Ricerche Farmacologiche Mario Negri, Milan.

Sian Griffiths is Director of Public Health and Health Policy at Oxfordshire Health Authority, Oxford.

Chris Ham is Director of the Health Services Management Centre at the University of Birmingham, Birmingham.

Søren Holm is Reader in Bioethics at the Centre for Social Ethics and Policy, University of Manchester, Manchester and Member of the Danish Council of Ethics.

Tony Hope is Lecturer in Practice Skills and Director of ETHOX at the Division of Public Health and Primary Healthcare at the University of Oxford.

Avi Israeli is Director General of the Hadassah Medical Organization, Jerusalem.

Kausar Khan is Assistant Professor in the Department of Community Health Sciences at The Aga Khan University, Karachi.

Rudolf Klein is Senior Associate at the King's Fund, London.

Boaz Lev is Deputy Director General for Medical Services and Quality Assurance at the Ministry of Health, Jerusalem.

Douglas K. Martin is Research Associate at the University of Toronto Joint Centre for Bioethics, Toronto.

Penelope Mullen is Senior Lecturer at the Health Services Management Centre, University of Birmingham, Birmingham.

Ole Frithjof Norheim is Associate Professor at the Division of General Practice, University of Bergen, Bergen.

Jorma Palo is Professor of Neurology in the Department of Clinical Neurosciences at the University of Helsinki, Helsinki.

Bryan Parry is Professor and Head of Department in the Department of Surgery at the Faculty of Medicine and Health Science, University of Auckland.

John Reynolds is Clinical Pharmacologist at the Oxford Radcliffe, Oxford.

James Sabin is Associate Director at the Harvard Pilgrim Health Care, Harvard Medical School, Boston MA.

Carmel Shalev is Director of the Unit for Health Rights and Ethics, Gertner Health Policy Institute, Tel Hashomer.

Peter Singer is Sun Life Chair in Bioethics and Director of the University of Toronto Joint Centre for Bioethics and a Medical Research Council of Canada Scientist.

Alan Williams is Professor in the Centre for Health Economics at the University of York, York.

John R. Williams is Director of Ethics at the Canadian Medical Association, Ottawa.

Michael Yeo is an Ethicist at the Canadian Medical Association, Ottawa.

SERIES EDITOR'S INTRODUCTION

Health services in many developed countries have come under critical scrutiny in recent years. In part this is because of increasing expenditure, much of it funded from public sources, and the pressure this has put on governments seeking to control public spending. Also important has been the perception that resources allocated to health services are not always deployed in an optimal fashion. Thus at a time when the scope for increasing expenditure is extremely limited, there is a need to search for ways of using existing budgets more efficiently. A further concern has been the desire to ensure access to health care of various groups on an equitable basis. In some countries this has been linked to a wish to enhance patient choice and to make service providers more responsive to patients as 'consumers'.

Underlying these specific concerns are a number of more fundamental developments which have a significant bearing on the performance of health services. Three are worth highlighting. First, there are demographic changes, including the ageing population and the decline in the proportion of the population of working age. These changes will both increase the demand for health care and at the same time limit the ability of health services to respond to this demand.

Second, advances in medical science will also give rise to new demands within the health services. These advances cover a range of possibilities, including innovations in surgery, drug therapy, screening and diagnosis. The pace of innovation quickened as the end of the century approached, with significant implications for the funding and provision of services.

Third, public expectations of health services are rising as those who use services demand higher standards of care. In part, this is stimulated by developments within the health service, including the availability of new technology. More fundamentally, it stems from the emergence of a more educated and informed population, in which people are accustomed to being treated as consumers rather than patients.

Against this background, policy makers in a number of countries are reviewing the future of health services. Those countries which have traditionally relied on a market in health care are making greater use of regulation and planning. Equally, those countries which have traditionally relied on regulation and planning are moving towards a more competitive approach. In no country is there complete satisfaction with existing methods of financing and delivery, and everywhere there is a search for new policy instruments.

The aim of this series is to contribute to debate about the future of health services through an analysis of major issues in health policy. These issues have been chosen because they are both of current interest and of enduring importance. The series is intended to be accessible to students and informed lay readers as well as to specialists working in this field. The aim is to go beyond a textbook approach to health policy analysis and to encourage authors to move debate about their issue forward. In this sense, each book presents a summary of current research and thinking, and an exploration of future policy directions.

Professor Chris Ham
Director of Health Services Management Centre,
University of Birmingham

1

INTRODUCTION: INTERNATIONAL EXPERIENCE OF RATIONING (OR PRIORITY SETTING)

Chris Ham and Angela Coulter

Rationing or priority setting in health care is inevitable. Market-based systems ration access to care on the basis of people's ability to pay, or at least to acquire health insurance. The well-known failures of markets in health care, not least the failure to ensure access to necessary medical assistance for all citizens, have led governments in developed countries to intervene to regulate the funding and provision of health services. In most OECD countries, this has resulted in legislation to guarantee universal population coverage and to ensure that the services available are more or less comprehensive.

In regulated health care systems, responsibility for rationing is shared by politicians, managers and clinicians. Traditionally, it has been doctors' decisions that have played the major part in shaping access to treatment by patients, and these decisions have usually been made implicitly in the privacy of doctors' consulting rooms. Implicit decision making has come under pressure in the face of resource constraints and rising patient expectations. This has led politicians in a number of countries to address the challenge of rationing more explicitly by setting up committees and expert groups.

Before summarizing the experience of these countries, it is important to be clear about the way in which the word rationing is used in this book. Rationing has a variety of connotations and, as at the beginning of this Introduction, is often used interchangeably with the term priority setting. While some authors prefer to use rationing to refer only to decisions that affect individual patients (Klein *et al*. 1996), in our view it has come to be employed to describe the variety of ways in which choices in health care are made whether they affect individuals, communities or countries. There seems little point in view of this in drawing hard and fast distinctions between rationing and priority setting. It is for this reason that throughout this book the terms are used synonymously to refer to the allocation of resources in health care both in terms of the relative priority to be attached to different demands and needs and to decisions that are made not to fund treatment for individuals or groups.

The experience of some of those countries that have rationed health care explicitly is summarized in Box 1.1. What this illustrates is the range of approaches that have been taken and the wide variety of different systems in which explicit priority setting is on the agenda. As a recent review of international experience concluded, the clear message from the work that has been done is that

> there are no simple or technical solutions to the priority setting dilemma. The work carried out in Oregon, the Netherlands, New Zealand, Sweden and the UK can be likened to an exercise in policy learning in which policy makers have tried out a range of methods and approaches and have adjusted course several times in the process. What is also apparent is that explicit priority setting is a continuous process which is not amenable to 'once and for all' solutions. To use a sporting metaphor, it is more like a marathon than a sprint, and those systems that have recognised this, like Oregon and New Zealand, have put in place mechanisms to ensure that the issues involved are kept under continuous review.
>
> (Ham 1997: 63)

Box 1.1 International experience of priority setting

In Oregon a Health Services Commission was appointed in 1989 to make recommendations on how Medicaid coverage could be expanded to groups in the population previously excluded and how priorities could be set within the Medicaid programme. After testing a number of methods, the Commission drew on the results of public consultation, research evidence, professional opinion and the judgement of its members

Box 1.1 *cont.*

to draw up a list of around 700 pairs of conditions and treatments to be given priority for funding. Following adjustments required by the federal government to avoid discrimination against disabled people, the Oregon health plan was implemented in 1994 with 565 out of 696 treatments on the final priority list being funded. Since then the Commission has kept the list under review, adding mental health and chemical dependency services into the basic health care package and moving treatments up and down the list in the light of experience. As a consequence, enrolment in Medicaid has increased by over 100,000 and the basic package has been expanded to provide a full range of services.

In New Zealand a Core Services Committee was set up by the government in 1992 to advise on the basic health care package to be funded in that country's health care system. The Committee argued that setting priorities by drawing up a simple list of services was not appropriate and instead it made recommendations on the services it felt should receive higher priority and initiated a series of consensus conferences to draw up guidelines on particular treatments or conditions. The Committee was subsequently renamed the National Health Committee and in its more recent work it has focused particularly on promoting the use of evidence-based guidelines and developing clinical criteria to determine access to a number of elective surgical procedures. In so doing, the Committee has sought to consult the public and representatives of patients' interests as well as to involve doctors and other experts in its work.

In the Netherlands the report of the Dunning Committee, published in 1991, offered advice to the Dutch government on the determination of priorities in the reformed social insurance system. A comprehensive approach was proposed including an investment in health technology assessment, the use of guidelines and protocols, and the development of criteria to determine access to waiting lists and priority on waiting lists. The Committee also set out a framework of values and principles intended to assist decision makers to decide which services should be in the basic health care package. The framework entailed asking whether the service concerned was

Box 1.1 *cont.*

necessary, effective, efficient, and whether it could be left to personal responsibility. Underpinning the Dunning Committee's approach was a belief that explicit priority setting, including the exclusion of certain services, was necessary if access to essential care was to be guaranteed for all. The Dutch government has used this approach to stimulate debate about priority setting but on the whole has chosen not to exclude whole categories of care from funding.

In Sweden the Parliamentary Priorities Commission was appointed in 1992 to advise on how priorities should be set in that country's health care system. A discussion document was published in 1993 and a final report was issued in 1995. Both documents were influenced by the work of the Lonning Commission in Norway. What was distinctive about the Swedish approach was a membership drawn from all political parties, an emphasis on an ethical platform for setting priorities, and the elucidation of priority categories for use at both the policy and clinical levels of decision making. This did not result in recommendations for the exclusion of particular services or treatments but rather a way of thinking about priority setting to assist those responsible for taking decisions.

In the United Kingdom a working party on priority setting established under the joint sponsorship of the government, the Academy of Medical Royal Colleges, the British Medical Association and the National Association of Health Authorities and Trusts reported in 1997. The working party concluded that priority setting was inevitable and that work was required to ensure that this was widely understood. It proposed that there should be a debate about the values that should inform priority setting and training for those with responsibilities in this area. The government has supported health authorities by funding work through the research and development programme, including work on health technology assessment, clinical guidelines and systematic reviews on the effectiveness of medical interventions. The establishment of the National Institute for Clinical Excellence in 1999 will enable this work to be coordinated and in the longer term may provide the focus for work on priority setting at a national level of the kind found in other countries.

What then are the lessons that emerge from experience so far? First, it is clear that responsibility for rationing rests at a number of levels in regulated health care systems (see Box 1.2). At the macro level, politicians determine the level of funding to be allocated to the health services and how this should be distributed between areas and services. At the meso level, intermediate bodies such as sickness funds, health authorities and insurance companies make decisions on the allocation of resources to particular forms of treatment. At the micro level, clinicians use their judgement and experience to decide which patients should receive treatment and how much should be done for individual patients. Each level impacts on the others, with clinicians retaining considerable discretion, even though politicians and managers at the macro and meso levels have increasingly questioned implicit decision making.

Box 1.2 Levels of priority setting

1 Macro: the level of funding to be allocated to health services
2 The distribution of the budget between geographical areas and services
3 The allocation of resources to particular forms of treatment
4 The choice of which patients should receive access to treatment
5 Decisions on how much to spend on individual patients

Source: Klein (1993a)

A second lesson is that explicit rationing at all levels involves both the use of techniques and the application of judgement. A wide variety of techniques have been deployed ranging from analysis of the cost-effectiveness of different treatments to systematic reviews of the evidence on clinical outcomes and the adoption of scoring systems to rank priority for treatment. While all of these techniques have made a contribution to decision making, the shortcomings of technical approaches have also been exposed. This was most apparent in Oregon where the original attempt to use economic analysis was abandoned when gaps in data produced anomalous results in the ranking of treatments. Subsequently, members of the Oregon Health Services Commission used their judgement, informed by research-based evidence, expert opinion and values expressed by the public, to make recommendations on priorities for funding. In so doing, they were responding to the limitations of existing techniques for comparing the costs and benefits of alternative interventions and the lack of a common currency for choosing between these alternatives.

A third lesson follows, namely the importance of determining whose judgement is used in rationing. While the views and advice of medical and other experts are drawn on extensively, there is increasing interest in widening the debate to include the public and patients' representatives. Again, a range of methods have been deployed to understand the values and preferences of the public and patients (see Box 1.3). In some cases, these methods have been

---

Box 1.3 Public involvement in rationing

Public involvement in rationing has taken a number of forms. In the Netherlands, an extensive period of public consultation followed publication of the Dunning Committee's report. About 60 organizations were involved in discussions on choices in health care. These started in 1991 and ended in 1995. An evaluation of the process concluded that the public discussions reached about one-third of the population. As a consequence, there were changes in public opinion. For example, in 1990, 55 per cent of the population believed that all treatments must be available irrespective of cost, whereas in 1994 this had fallen to 44 per cent. Less positively, the results of the exercise were not used by the Dutch government in its decision-making process on choices in health care.

In Sweden, the work of the Parliamentary Priorities Commission was guided by a number of surveys of the public and of health care professionals. The survey of the public was carried out by questionnaire in January 1994, and involved a random sample of 1500 people. A 78 per cent response rate was achieved. A majority of respondents felt that medical care should be mainly devoted to people with the severest illnesses. A majority of respondents also agreed with the commission's recommendation that terminal care should be given the same high priority as emergency health care. Services that the public felt might be restricted included cosmetic surgery, removing harmless birthmarks, smoking cessation

Box 1.3 *cont.*

programmes and *in vitro* fertilization. Overall, the question-naire survey strongly endorsed the principles set out in the commission's first report.

In Oregon, the methods used included public hearings, community meetings and telephone surveys. An organization known as Oregon Health Decisions was commissioned to help with this work. Focus groups involved participants drawn from different sections of the community in discussing some of the choices that had to be made. Oregon Health Decisions concluded that this was a particularly effective way of extracting information from the community about values. Because of the small numbers involved, however, it was less effective as a method of engaging the community at large.

In New Zealand the National Health Committee undertook two major community consultation exercises early in its existence designed to find out the public's views on what health services the public valued and how the committee should decide what services should be publicly funded. A mixture of methods was used including town hall meetings and facilitated workshops with particular community groups. The committee has also used other methods including consensus conferences, *hui* and *fono* with Maori and Pacific Island communities, workshops, symposia, public forums, contestable expert advisory hearings, and meetings with groups which represent specific consumer interests. These face-to-face methods were supplemented by written communications of various kinds. Notwithstanding this, it is recognized that more needs to be done to promote patient and public involvement.

In the United Kingdom public involvement takes place mainly at a local level. Health authorities have used a variety of methods including questionnaire surveys, focus groups, health panels and public meetings. A number of innovations in democratic practice have also been employed, such as citizens' juries. In some cases these methods have been used to gather information about the public's views and values to inform decision making, whereas in others they have been part of an attempt to stimulate greater public understanding of rationing.

used to educate and inform citizens about the need for rationing; in others they have helped to identify the values the public feel are important in making decisions. In addition, consultation with patients and the organizations representing their views has contributed a user perspective to the rationing of particular services. The effort put into public and patient involvement follows from the attempt to make rationing more explicit and to extend the circle of participants beyond those in formal decision-making roles at the macro, meso and micro levels.

Fourth, attempts to be more explicit about rationing have revealed the difficulty of defining a basic basket of services or benefits package by excluding some treatments from funding. Oregon did go down this route and decided to restrict the services to be funded under Medicaid (the government-funded programme of health care for people on low incomes) in order to include more people within the scope of this programme. Elsewhere, those charged with responsibility for rationing have usually declined to draw up a list of core services, focusing instead on ensuring that the full range of services are provided to those who can benefit most from them. This was the approach taken in New Zealand by the government-appointed Core Services Committee which offered the following justification for its approach:

> One of the first things the committee did decide was that the core could not simply be a list of services, treatments or conditions that would or would not receive public funding . . . The approach we decided to take was one that has flexibility to take account of an individual's circumstances when deciding if a service or treatment should be publicly funded. For example . . . instead of a decision that says hormone replacement therapy (HRT) is either core or non-core . . . the committee has decided that in certain circumstances HRT will be a core service and in others it won't be. The committee has recommended that HRT be a core service where there is clinical and research based agreement that it constitutes an appropriate and effective treatment. Where such agreement does not exist, or where evidence or indications make its use inappropriate, then HRT should not be funded from the public purse.
>
> (Jones 1993)

The strength of these arguments is reinforced by evidence that attempts to exclude services generate opposition from the groups affected. This has been the case in the Netherlands, for example in relation to a proposal that contraceptive pills should no longer be available free at the point of use, and this explains why, in that country,

> decisions on the form of the basic benefits package have rarely sought to exclude entire groups of services, but have tended to restrict these services at the fringes by limiting the extent to which the service is covered. For example, women under 40 years of age *are* entitled to *in vitro* fertilisation, but to no more than three interventions.
>
> (Dunning 1996)

A fifth lesson which follows on from the difficulty of 'rationing by exclusion' (Ham 1995) is that setting priorities by drawing up guidelines for the provision of services has attracted increasing interest. In the case of New Zealand, the committee charged with responsibility for rationing has placed particular emphasis on the use of consensus conferences, bringing together experts and lay people to make recommendations on the guidelines that should be adopted for treatments such as the management of raised blood pressure and end-stage kidney failure. New Zealand has also established a programme of work on the development and implementation of guidelines under the aegis of the Core Services Committee (since renamed the National Health Committee). Similarly, rationing in the Netherlands has focused on the development of guidelines by professional associations as the debate in that country has moved away from restricting the scope of the benefits package through political decisions at the macro level to ensuring that resources are used efficiently by clinicians at the micro level. Much the same applies in the United Kingdom where successive governments have rejected the idea that national lists of treatments should be defined and instead have encouraged the development of clinical guidelines, supporting this work by funding expert groups to undertake health technology assessments.

Sixth, the emphasis placed on evidence-based guidelines as a mechanism of rationing is part of a much wider movement to strengthen the scientific basis of medicine. This has found expression in the establishment of agencies on health technology assessment in a number of countries and in the concern to reduce variations in clinical practice patterns. Both politicians and managers have been at the forefront of these efforts, challenging clinical freedom in the pursuit of continuous improvements in efficiency and quality. In the process, the limits of what has been described as the 'new scientism'

(Klein *et al.* 1996) have also been exposed as analysts have pointed to medical uncertainty and limitations in the evidence base as constraints on the attempt to make priority setting at the micro level more scientific. Notwithstanding these constraints, the momentum behind the evidence-based medicine movement continues to increase as strategies to manage clinical activity gain support in health services with quite different systems of financing and delivery.

A seventh and rather different lesson is that the emphasis on judgement in arriving at decisions has drawn attention to the role of values in rationing. This is because the relative priority attached to different types of treatments or services (for example, to palliative care for the terminally ill as opposed to intensive care for those with life-threatening conditions) depends in part on the value attached to different outcomes (such as improving the quality of life as opposed to increasing the length of life). Information about values gathered from the public can help to inform judgements of this kind and ensure that they are not based solely on the advice of experts or the preferences of decision makers. The need to make these kinds of choices illustrates the ethical dilemmas involved in rationing and the moral basis of decision making. These ethical dilemmas have been addressed in a number of countries including Sweden where the committee appointed to advise on rationing proposed an ethical platform centred on respect for human dignity, equity and efficiency as a basis for making choices. Other countries have adopted different values (Ham 1997), illustrating the inherently contested nature of this debate.

An eighth and final lesson is the increasing interest shown in the process of decision making. In the absence of technical solutions to rationing problems, the way in which priorities are set has been seen as an important element in the task of securing legitimacy for decisions which in many circumstances may be both controversial and unpopular. The focus on the decision-making process is of course related to the interest in explicit rationing and to the attempt to involve the public and patients in debate on these issues. It is also linked to rising demands and expectations on the part of service users and the decline of deference to health care professionals, particularly at a time when resource constraints reinforce the suspicion that decisions not to fund treatments may be based on financial rather than clinical considerations. One reaction has been to seek to make decision making more transparent and consistent and to allow opportunities for patients and their families to appeal against decisions. This is seen at least in part as a way of promoting wider deliberation and understanding of priority setting at a time when both public and media interest in this field is increasing, not least in response to individual cases that have come to epitomize the challenge of making tragic choices in health care (Ham and Pickard 1998).

LEARNING FROM EXPERIENCE

To highlight these lessons is to underline the point made at the outset that international experience of rationing has been an exercise in policy learning involving trial and error and a testing of different approaches. That the exercise is continuing is illustrated by the increasing number of countries (Israel and Denmark being two recent examples) exploring more explicit and systematic approaches and the burgeoning literature in this field (as examples see New 1997 and Lenaghan 1997). Another indication of the strength of interest is the plethora of meetings and conferences on rationing, including a number with a comparative focus. In the present context, of particular note was the staging of the first international conference on priorities in health care in Stockholm in 1996 followed by a second conference in London in 1998.

The chapters in this book were selected from papers presented at the London conference and they offer a selective summary of work in progress in different countries. They have been chosen to reflect experience in various parts of the world as well as to shed light on some of the themes that have emerged from experience. In presenting them here we make no claim to their representativeness nor to complete coverage of the field. What is clear is that they have been written by authors deeply involved in rationing as researchers or practitioners and with experience that holds lessons for others.

The rest of the book is divided into seven sections with chapters giving different viewpoints on specific topics. Rationing is a contentious subject. Even when there is consensus about its inevitability, there remains considerable debate about how it should be done. This debate is reflected in the contributions to the book. Chapter 2 opens up the issues with a debate between Alan Williams, a leading proponent of the need to ration explicitly by using quantitative techniques such as QALYs to decide between competing priorities, and Rudolf Klein, who takes a sceptical view of the usefulness of formal approaches to the problem.

The next four chapters describe approaches to rationing adopted by governments in the Nordic countries, Israel and the USA. As Søren Holm explains in Chapter 3, the early optimism about the possibility of finding simple solutions to the problem has given way to a focus on the process itself, with attempts to ensure that decision making is transparent, inclusive and accountable.

Developing countries face even starker choices and these are the subject of Chapters 7 and 8 which both draw on experience in Pakistan. As Kausar Khan points out, health is a fundamental human right and the needs of poor people need to be given greater priority by national governments than is sometimes the case.

Whatever the setting, decision makers in the health care field face difficult ethical choices. The work of the American philosopher Norman Daniels has been influential among those involved in rationing. He describes his approach in Chapter 9 and his theme is taken up by the authors of the following three chapters.

The search for better techniques to allocate health care resources continues. Chapter 13 outlines different approaches which have been developed and Chapter 14 describes New Zealand clinicians' experiences of using scoring systems to determine who should be admitted from the waiting list.

Techniques for increasing public involvement in rationing are the subject of the following section. Chapter 15 critically reviews various methods and Chapters 16 and 17 describe experience of putting some of these into practice.

Ultimately resource use in most countries is determined by the decisions and treatment choices made by individual clinicians and their patients. Governments and local health authorities have made various attempts to influence these choices to ensure equitable and cost-effective distribution of resources. The next section includes three chapters which describe attempts to support and shape clinical decision making in Britain, Italy and Norway. The experience in these and other countries underlines the point that clinical decision making can never be a purely technical exercise – people's values, beliefs and preferences exert a crucial influence on the choices that are made.

The final chapter returns to the issues introduced here, pulling together the diverse experiences reported in the contributions from different countries to identify some common themes and to highlight areas for further research and debate.

PART I

HOW TO SET PRIORITIES

2

SETTING PRIORITIES: WHAT IS HOLDING US BACK – INADEQUATE INFORMATION OR INADEQUATE INSTITUTIONS?

Rudolf Klein and Alan Williams

This chapter is based on material used in a debate at the 1998 International Conference on Priorities in Health Care in which Alan Williams argued that inadequate information was the main problem, and Rudolf Klein argued that the main problem was inadequate institutions. What we have done here is first to repeat our original arguments, after which each of us comments on the views of the other. So this chapter falls into four sections: Williams's original case; Klein's original case; Williams's response; and Klein's response. There is no summing up – readers are left to make up their own minds on which way the balance of the argument goes!

WILLIAMS'S CASE: A LITTLE MORE THOUGHT BEFORE ANY FURTHER ACTION

I start from the assumption that effective priority setting requires clarity about objectives, information about costs and outcomes, and the ability to measure performance (since all health care systems are bound to be strongly decentralized). I will consider each of these in turn.

Clarity about objectives requires coherent thought at the centre, and clear messages flowing through the system. The rationale for the content of these messages needs to be evident to those receiving them, otherwise they are not likely to be strongly motivated to act upon them. That implies that comprehensible criteria for choice have been promulgated, and that the information necessary to apply these criteria is available to those charged with the responsibility of using them.

At a very general level, most health care systems have two broad objectives, which are:

- to improve population health; and
- to reduce inequalities in health

as much as possible with the resources available.

That sort of statement is fine at the centre, but before it can constitute any sort of guidance for those with operational responsibilities at lower levels, a great deal of clarification is required.

First, which population are we talking about? Is it just current patients? Or does it also include those known to be waiting for treatment? Or does it widen out still more to include anyone who might ever become a patient? Is there a citizenship requirement or some other test of entitlement? Is responsibility restricted geographically? And so on.

Second, what is meant by health in this context? Is it to be a clinical biomedical measurement of disease or of symptom prevalence, or is it to concentrate on mortality and life expectancy, or widen its scope and look at self-reported health-related quality of life, such as mobility problems, or pain, or anxiety, or depression, or the ability to look after oneself without help? Each of these measures directs one's attention in a different direction, and hence will have a marked impact upon the kind of priorities that are set.

Third, are all inequalities equally reprehensible and of equal concern to public policy, or does it depend to some extent on how they are caused? What sacrifices should those who have cared for their own health be called upon to make for those who are suffering because they knowingly took risks with their health?

Fourth, what do we know about the values of the general public on all of these matters? Are health service professionals good proxies for the views of the general public, or do they have special interests of their own which might bias their judgements, wittingly or unwittingly?

Fifth, what are the appropriate resource constraints to take into account? Is it just the resources assigned to the particular decision maker, or should some regard also be paid to costs falling on the rest of the health care system? Or should the remit be wider still, so that costs falling on any public services need to be considered (which might be particularly important at the interface between health services and social support and social security)? Then there are the limited resources of the patients and their families to be thought about. What is the decision maker expected to do?

And sixth, what are to be the trade-offs between all these different desiderata when some conflict occurs between them? Two major strategic issues arise here. The first of these lies in the conflict between maximizing population health generally and reducing inequalities in health, where the classic equity–efficiency trade-off manifests itself. The second lies in the setting of a resource limit on what a particular health gain is worth (which is the essence of the priority-setting problem). This latter point is often wrapped up in the language of 'affordability', but what you can 'afford' depends both on your resources and on your priorities, and if these matters are both unclear, then so will be the affordability criterion. What is needed here is *thought* and *evidence* – no amount of institutional reform is going to resolve these issues (though some institutional reforms have the comfortable, but misplaced, property of hiding them from sight!).

Information about costs and outcomes remains a problem even when the conceptual issues mentioned above have been resolved satisfactorily. But the problem is greatly exacerbated at present because there is very muddled thinking about objectives, so that outcome measurement degenerates rather quickly into measuring anything that moves! Thus, measures of activity usurp the role that measures of health gain should be playing, and the output of the system is taken to be the number of people treated, or the available bed-days. This leads us into the dangerous fallacy of believing that more means better.

Then, to lend respectability to that position, the objectives of the system get transformed into statements such as

- to provide health care for the population;
- to ensure equal access to health care.

The contrast between these two objectives and the two stated earlier is revealing. Priority setting then becomes emasculated, because testing performance against these two objectives requires no measurement of health gain whatever! But without data on costs and benefits and who will enjoy them, how are we to choose between the claims of rival service providers for the scarce resources? And is not accessibility instrumental, rather than an end in itself? If the objective is indeed to reduce inequalities in *health* then it may be necessary to have deliberately unequal *accessibility* so as to favour the worse off.

Paradoxically, the present lack of information about outcomes is often used as a justification for using these process measures instead, when it should be being used as a justification for redirecting effort towards filling the vacuum. And since many outcome measures are currently rather crude and approximate compared with the more familiar process measures, they are often set aside for this reason too. But surely it is better to get the important things approximately right than to get the wrong things measured accurately! Again it is a case where *thought* and *evidence* are needed, rather than yielding the field of play to *intellectual inertia*.

The situation on the cost side is not a great deal better, for reasons mentioned earlier. There is heavy reliance on the routine financial system to generate suitable data on the costs of achieving health gains in different ways. But it was never designed for this purpose, and it is ill-equipped to fulfil it. It was designed to ensure that money only got spent in legitimate ways on the things it was intended to be spent on. It is essentially a control system, not an evaluation system. It can provide information on how much was paid to whom for what, but it cannot tell us routinely whether those goods or services could have been obtained more cheaply, nor whether they were really needed at all, nor whether they did the job they were supposed to do. And because the financial system is there to track the currently available money through the system, it gives us very little guidance on the use of assets that were bought earlier, or on things which the health service gets without having to pay for them.

The most important of these 'free' resources is the use of patients' time, which does have an opportunity cost even though the health service does not meet it. Thus patients' time is used profligately by the system, as any 'free' resource would be, yet when appraising the efficiency of a system, and determining priorities, we would not want to emulate the financial system and regard patients' time as worthless. This major difference between economics (which looks at all resources that have value to people) and finance (which looks only at resources that cost money) is at the heart of much of the misunderstanding that surrounds the role of costs in priority setting. People who should know better think that a concern about costs is simply a concern about money. To an economist it is a concern about the sacrifices that people are being called upon to make, in terms of the other things they value that have to be given up.

Performance measurement requires that all this information be summarized into operationally meaningful criteria that flow directly from the general objectives of the system. This means that the information system that supports priority setting must concentrate on costs and outcomes rather than on cash and activity levels, relevant though these are at an instrumental level in seeing who is doing what to whom. But we need also to answer the question, 'With what effect?' (in terms of health gain) and, 'Instead of what?' (to get some idea of the sacrifices in health gain imposed on others). Managerial 'targets' are typically directed at activity levels, and we shall know when the performance of the system has become more closely related to its ostensible objectives when someone is fired or demoted for failing to deliver enough health gain to the population served!

If those problems are endemic even for the more straightforward objective of improving the population's health as much as possible, how much more intractable they appear to be when it comes to the objective of reducing inequalities in health. In many health care systems it seems to be believed that if resources are equalized between different parts of the system on some population-weighted basis, then the problem of reducing inequalities in health has been dealt with, but this is patently not the case. For one thing, there is no guarantee that the resources provided will be used to reduce inequalities in health, and it is rare to find performance measures designed to check on this. What would be needed is routine data on population health which addresses inequalities directly (for instance by measuring quality-adjusted life expectancy at various ages, and identifying the causes of the great differences that exist within populations, even in countries which are proud of their egalitarian ethos). Once again there is a great gap between the political rhetoric emanating from the centre of most systems, and the measurement of performance at the operational level.

So what is to be done about all this? Wringing our hands in despair is understandable, but not very helpful except as an indicator that we do see that there is a problem. It will not be an easy task to fill the vacuum, and in the short run the results will not be spectacular. What is required is a major shift of thinking *and resources* towards the kind of outcome measurement required for strategic priority setting, and the adoption of economic appraisal techniques as the standard evaluative method for all health care activities. If half the resources that have been devoted to institutional reform had been devoted to this task instead, priority setting would now have a much better evidence base than it actually has, and without such a shift we shall be facing the same difficulties in ten years' time as we are facing now.

One of the main obstacles to progress is the clash of cultures between analysts who see the need for clarity and openness, and politicians (including the professional wielders of power within the health care system) who rightly feel vulnerable when their muddled thinking and inadequate evidence base are exposed to external scrutiny. And since their authority derives partly from their claim to be accountable to the public, this exposure is particularly dangerous.

So although we are treated to a great deal of rhetoric about public accountability and consumer involvement, this is not matched by any real commitment to provide the missing evidence about cost-effectiveness on which any well-informed involvement would depend. But since something has to be seen to be being done, what better response could there be than institutional reform? It is dramatic, it gets widely reported, it distracts everyone from thinking about the fundamental problems, and is the modern equivalent of providing circuses for the masses in place of bread. And since it takes some time for things to shake down again, it takes some time for people to realize that they still have to confront the problem of priority setting, for which they still don't have clarity of objectives, nor data on costs and outcomes, nor appropriate performance measures! But by then the politicians have changed and the new ones are dreaming up some other organizational reform to keep the system in a permanent state of muddle. And the talent that could have been devoted to dealing with the inescapable fundamentals is diverted once more into superficialities!

I rest my case.

KLEIN'S CASE: WHY INSTITUTIONS MATTER MORE THAN INFORMATION

My initial proposition is simple. It is that, given conflicting values, the process of setting priorities for health care must inevitably be a process of debate. It is a debate, moreover, which cannot be resolved by an appeal to science and where the search for some formula or set of principles designed to provide decision-making rules will always prove elusive. Hence the crucial importance of getting the *institutional* setting of the debate right: of ensuring that the debate will not be dominated by one particular interest (e.g. the medical profession) and that all voices can make themselves heard. I am not arguing that getting the process right will necessarily provide the 'right' answers. I do not think that in the context of setting health care priorities there is necessarily a 'right' answer, independent of an ever-shifting context. My contention is less ambitious: it is that the right process will produce socially acceptable answers – and that this is the best we can hope for.

Let me justify these assertions. The foundation of my argument is that there is no one value or principle from which we can derive our health care priorities. Is this right? What about maximizing the health of the population? Does this not trump other possible values or principles – such as the rule of rescue? I don't think so. Even if we accept the utilitarian approach, 'maximizing the health of the population' is after all a second-order principle. The presumption is that it serves the first-order principle of maximizing the welfare of the population. But what if the two conflict? What if the welfare of the population (its sense of security and solidarity) is maximized by a collective willingness to undertake heroic rescues that, on a narrow health-based utilitarian calculus, appear to be a nonsense?

Again, there seems to be much support for the view that in the queue for resources the young should be given priority over the elderly. Here, surely, we have got the kind of agreed principle that can help us to shape health care priorities. But have we? No doubt Alan Williams and I, old age pensioners both, would agree that money should not be spent on us to prolong the last few months of our lives with heroic interventions and that we should not have high priority for heart transplants. However, concentrating on expensive interventions oversimplifies the real policy issues in setting health care priorities. Many of these have nothing to do with high-tech drama and everything to do with providing support and relief for long-standing chronic conditions. If we took 'maximizing the ability of people to lead normal lives and play their role in society' as our guiding principle in determining resource allocation, might this not tilt expenditure towards the elderly?

The case of using age as a priority-setting discriminator raises a wider issue. Different considerations may come into play, depending on whether the issue involved is about rationing access to a particular package of resources or about determining the distribution of those resources in the first place. Even if we agree that age can be used as an acceptable proxy discriminator when deciding on prioritizing access to a particular treatment (e.g. renal dialysis), it is much less useful as a guide to decision making about the distribution of resources between different sectors of health care and the level and quality of health care that should be delivered within them.

I could go on about the problems that arise when we try to find and apply appropriate principles to particular issues. The case of *in vitro* fertilization (IVF) would provide rich text, raising the question of the social construction of 'medical necessity'. However, I think I have made my point. Priority setting is about policy making, not just about devising neat academic formulae. And the problems of policy making do not stem primarily from a lack of information, but from a lack of consensus about how to use and interpret it. Of course, more information is always desirable, but we should be aware that it often speaks with forked tongues and that it may outstrip our capacity to master it. Moreover, the most relevant information may be that generated by the policy process itself: i.e. how particular decisions about priorities (and the criteria used) work out in practice. Indeed, the evidence generated by the policy process may, in turn, affect preferences as the consequences, both anticipated and unanticipated, emerge. The weight given to competing values or principles implicit in priority setting may thus change over time.

Which brings me to my conclusion. The strategy of advocating continuing debate, and designing institutions that will promote it, is often presented as a retreat from rationality. Instead of advancing boldly on to the intellectual heights in search of the philosopher's stone – basing policy on a body of incontrovertible 'facts' that point ineluctably towards a specific conclusion – it seems to be no more than 'muddling through'. I would suggest that, on the contrary, it represents a more sophisticated version of rationality than the naïve form of rationality which assumes that more information and better analysis are the answer. More sophisticated because it recognizes – as Braybrooke and Lindblom showed us a long time ago – that policy making is inevitably a process of trial and error ('disjointed incrementalism' they called it) where rationality lies in the willingness to learn from experience. And one of the most valuable contributions of cross-national comparisons and explorations will be what it tells us about this process: what we can learn from the experience of different countries and different policy makers when trying to set priorities.

WILLIAMS'S RESPONSE

It appears that from the same starting point Klein and I reach very different conclusions! I agree that 'given conflicting values, the process of setting priorities for health care must inevitably be a process of debate', and if by 'resolved' he means 'solved' I also agree that it 'cannot be resolved by an appeal to science'. I also agree that 'the search for some formula or set of principles designed to provide decision-making rules will also prove elusive'. But from these observations Klein concludes that we can dispense with 'the naïve form of rationality which assumes that more information and better analysis are the answer' and replace it with 'a more sophisticated version' 'where rationality lies in the willingness to learn by experience'.

This distinction has me puzzled. How do we 'learn from experience' except by gathering information and analysing it carefully? And how is this to be a purposive activity unless guided by some set of principles which reflects our best understanding of what we are trying to achieve? Policy making is undoubtedly a process of trial and error, but it should not be done by blindfolded people taking pot-shots randomly in whatever direction they happen to be facing! In health care reform we have witnessed far too much innovation without evaluation. Sometimes it is driven by ideological beliefs in the inherent merits of, say, markets as opposed to planning (or vice versa), which are held not to require evidence to be collected or analysed. Sometimes it is driven by the belief that the grass seems greener over there, so why don't we do what they are doing so that our grass will be greener too. When, eventually, it has to be admitted that such an innovation has patently failed to deliver what was anticipated, some fresh 'stunt' has to be dreamed up to maintain the political momentum. But since no proper analysis can be done (because of lack of evidence) to identify why the previous one failed, this next innovation will be a shot in the dark too! If this is what 'sophisticated rationality' is all about, I think the sooner we go back to the more naïve version the better.

Surely 'learning by experience' requires every innovation to be approached in a more scientific frame of mind, in which the criteria of success or failure are specified *ex ante*, and systematically related to the objectives that are being pursued. A plan of evaluation needs to be devised and implemented so that we can not only see whether the innovation is working as expected, but if not, why not! That is a difficult thing to do, but without it the learning capacity of the system is severely limited. Indeed, all you may learn is that X misled us all and had better be thrown out, only to be replaced by Y who, if another 'sophisticated muddler', may well lead us up a different garden path with similarly disastrous results!

Perhaps it is the distrust of systematic evaluative thinking that distinguishes politicians, and some political scientists too it seems, from economists and other empirically based social scientists on the one hand, and from doctors and the public health community on the other, all of whom accept the need to collect and analyse evidence as the most important means of learning by doing. Perhaps it is time to start a crusade for evidence-based politics!

KLEIN'S RESPONSE

Let me start, like Alan Williams, by identifying an area of agreement. We agree that it would be highly desirable to improve the quality of thought and analysis that informs health policy making at all levels and on all issues, including the setting of priorities. On that point there is no dispute. The reason why I give primacy to institutions, as against information, is that unless we strengthen our *institutional capacity* to analyse evidence, to clarify policy choices and to promote informed debate, generating more information is more likely to compound confusion than to lead to better decision making. At the level of clinical policy making, the creation of the National Institute for Clinical Excellence (NICE) can be seen as one step in this direction. At the level of national policy making, our institutional capacity remains weak. For example, the Health Committee of the House of Commons conspicuously lacks supporting expertise: there may be a case for linking it to the Audit Commission, in the same way that the National Audit Office supports the Public Accounts Committee. Similarly, while the research councils and the Department of Health's research and development (R & D) programme support research, policy analysis remains an academic orphan with the result that our collective ability to make use of the information that is available is inadequate. Nor is it self-evident that more information will necessarily improve the quality of debate in the media: a key issue where no easy solution is in sight. Hence the case for strengthening institutions before clamouring for more evidence.

In any case, to return to the theme of my opening statement, evidence may inform decision making about priorities but it cannot (and should not) determine the outcome. Only consider some of the policy dilemmas and muddles identified by Williams. Is our objective to maximize the population's health or to minimize inequalities? Are all inequalities equally reprehensible and of equal concern to public policy? No amount of evidence will answer these questions. If we want guidance we are more likely to look to social theorists than to economists: the arguments will hinge on societal values, not on evidence about cost-effectiveness.

The same point applies to decisions about rationing. In some cases, cost-effectiveness evidence may indeed be the clincher when it comes to deciding whether or not to make a particular procedure or drug available in the NHS. In other instances, very different considerations will apply. The case of Viagra – perhaps the first explicit, national rationing decision in the history of the National Health Service (NHS) – is a case in point. Here the Secretary of State's decision reflected his view that 'impotence is in itself neither life-threatening, nor does it cause physical pain'. In effect, therefore, the Secretary of State was redefining the remit of the NHS, limiting it by implication to dealing with conditions that threaten life or cause pain: a new principle. Whether right or wrong, the decision calls for analysis and debate about the implications of the principle for the way in which we think about the NHS's activities – drawing on our existing stock of knowledge rather than attempting to generate more evidence.

There is a danger, furthermore, in having too narrow a view of the nature of 'evidence' by invoking the name of 'science'. Economic appraisal techniques and randomized controlled trials (RCTs) are only one kind of evidence. They are useful for settling particular kinds of arguments if they provide clear-cut conclusions (which, very often, is not the case: the output may frequently be frustrating ambiguity). But there are other kinds of evidence. The political system – whatever its other weaknesses – is a powerful machine for generating evidence about the acceptability of public policies: a crucial consideration when it comes to deciding on priorities. The administrative machinery of the NHS is a mechanism for generating information about the way in which public policies are working out and for providing feedback to Ministers – and could be made more effective still if the information so generated were made more transparent (another argument for institutional reform).

Indeed, the notion that public policies should be designed in a way to make them fit for evaluation by the scientific community is faintly comic in its arrogance. Is it really conceivable that Ministers would stick to their policies regardless of the information generated by the political and administrative processes, rather than constantly adjusting them in the process of implementation in the light of the evidence that is landing on their desks? Should they really be sitting patiently awaiting the results of a formal evaluation, ignoring all the signals and information generated by the policy itself? And if they do (quite rightly) adapt policy goals and change policy instruments as they go along, how is an evolving, self-transforming target to be assessed? Further, one of the great problems of evaluation is making a sensible guess at the timescale needed for any policy to demonstrate its impact (or lack of it). Usually it is longer than the electoral cycle or the lifespan of individual Ministers.

The attempt to devise more 'rational' techniques of policy making has a long history, going back at least to the 1960s when a variety of new tools were imported from the United States: programme budgeting, programme analysis and review, and so on. Alan Williams was indeed a pioneer in promoting such techniques in this country. Yet, more than 30 years later, there is still the same despairing demand for more 'systematic evaluative thinking' and economists still think that their contribution to policy making is undervalued. Two explanations for this phenomenon of frustrated hopes and ambitions offer themselves. The first is that those who see themselves as the champions of rationality have failed in what should be their first analytical task, which is to understand the processes of policy making. The second is that they define rationality – and evidence – too narrowly and, it might be said, in a self-interested disciplinary way. And if their answer to these conclusions is that the political processes themselves ought to be changed – in order to create a policy universe fit for economists and those of a similar cast of mind – then that surely makes my point: that institutions have primacy over information.

PART II

GOVERNMENTS AND RATIONING

3

DEVELOPMENTS IN THE NORDIC COUNTRIES – GOODBYE TO THE SIMPLE SOLUTIONS

Søren Holm

Public health care systems in the Nordic countries share two key characteristics:

- funding is raised either through general taxation or through some form of compulsory contribution related to income but unrelated to disease state or use of the health care system
- the hospitals are publicly owned and managed.

These institutional features have shaped both the structure and the content of the Nordic debate about priorities in health care. Structurally it has meant that the debate has centred around a number of official reports published in these countries. With regard to content, the problems discussed have been the problems which plague most public health care systems: waiting lists, service of questionable quality, lack of choice between providers, etc. The debate began in earnest in the early 1980s and has in recent years been further intensified by economic stagnation in some of the Nordic countries.

In this chapter I will try to show that the debate can be viewed as consisting of two different phases: a first phase where the focus was on the outcome of priority setting, and a second phase where the focus has moved to the process of priority setting. Some of the Nordic countries are well into the transition to Phase 2, whereas others are still in Phase 1. The main features of the two phases are outlined in Box 3.1.

Box 3.1   Basic assumptions of the two phases of the priority-setting debates

Phase 1
- There is a principled way of making priority decisions and it is possible to devise a rational priority-setting system.
- Decisions made by applying the correct priority-setting system are *ipso facto* legitimate.

Phase 2
- There is no principled way of making priority decisions.
- Decisions made through the correct priority-setting process are *ipso facto* legitimate.
- The correct priority-setting process is characterized by transparency and accountability.

THE SEARCH FOR SOLUTIONS TO THE PRIORITY PROBLEM

When the debate about priorities in health care first began in the Nordic countries in the early 1980s, the stated goal was to find solutions to the priority-setting problems. Public awareness of growing waiting lists and demands for new kinds of services brought about a slow realization that choices would have to be made between different health care interventions. The need for priority setting had previously often been explicitly denied, and calls for a discussion even decried as unethical. In 1987 the first Norwegian report on priority setting in health care was published and it set the stage for the debate about this issue in the Nordic countries for a number of years (Norges Offentlige Utredninger 1987). Later the Dutch report of 1992 also had a major impact on the debate (Ministry of Welfare, Health and Cultural Affairs 1992).

The Norwegian report argued for a system based on five levels of priorities arranged according to the severity of the disease/condition in question and the consequences of not treating it. Similar schemes were later reproduced with minor modifications in the official Finnish report of 1994 and the official Swedish report of 1995 (STAKES 1994; Sveriges Offentliga Utredningar 1995).

Health economists complained that these priority-setting systems were misguided because they were based almost exclusively on severity of disease, and not on any kind of effectiveness measure, such as marginal expenditure per quality adjusted life year (QALY) gained for different kinds of treatment–condition pairs. The decision-making systems usually proposed by economists are very different (often some version of cost-utility or cost-benefit analysis), but they share one feature with the systems in the official reports. That is the belief that it is possible to design systems which can give definite answers to priority problems.

The first phase in discussions and reports about health care priorities was thus characterized by a search for priority-setting systems that, through a complete and non-contradictory set of rational decision rules, could tell the decision maker precisely how a given service should be prioritized vis-à-vis other services. Given appropriate information the priority-setting algorithm should be able to give determinate and compelling answers. These answers would be legitimate because they flowed from an objective and rational set of rules. Once agreement has been reached on the rules, and on the information fed into the system, there can be no disagreement about the legitimacy of the result, and no possibility for further discussion.

GOODBYE TO THE SIMPLE SOLUTIONS

The second phase of the debates about priority setting began to emerge in the early 1990s. It was first embodied and endorsed in an official report in 1996 when the Danish Council of Ethics published its final report on priority setting in the Danish health care system (Danish Council of Ethics 1996). This was followed in 1997 by a second Norwegian report on priorities, reflecting on the experiences with the system implemented after the 1987 report (Norges Offentlige Utredninger 1997).

The Danish Council argued that none of the priority-setting systems which had been produced were really operational, and all suffered from one or both of two fatal flaws:

- they were based on a simplistic view about the purpose of the health care system; and/or
- they did not really give any specific guidance as to how one should prioritize.

The Danish report argued that we cannot reduce the goal of a public health care system of the Nordic type to only one thing. A public health care system is not there simply to maximize the amount of health in society (however we choose to measure health). It is not there merely to treat diseases (however we choose to define disease). It is not there solely to meet health care needs (however we choose to define health care needs). And it is not there to ensure equality in health status (however we choose to concep-tualize equality). The goal of a public health care system is a com-plex composite of a range of goals, including more fuzzy goals like heightening the sense of security in the population. There is no nat-ural way to balance these goals against each other. We can state that one goal is more important than another in specific situations, but an attempt to elevate one goal as the most important in all situ-ations is simply implausible. In some priority-setting contexts relieving the largest amount of suffering is more important than equality, whereas in other contexts the opposite is the case. This means that it becomes impossible to use a simple maximizing algo-rithm as the basis for a priority-setting system (such an algorithm requires either a single goal, or a principled way of balancing a number of goals[1]).

The Danish Council of Ethics also pointed to other conceptual problems with the allegedly rational decision-making systems pro-posed during the first phase. These problems can be illustrated by looking at one of the most common allocation criteria mentioned during the first phase: the severity of the disease.[2] Initially it may seem that we know what we mean when we talk about the severity of a disease, but on closer analysis the concept of severity shows itself to be open to a variety of different interpretations. Whether or not a disease is lethal or likely to lead to permanent handicap or disability is an aspect of its severity (cancer is a severe disease, even if it does not cause any present symptoms). However, the concept of severity also includes the present health state, e.g. whether there is severe pain or present disability (shingles is a severe disease, even though it is of limited duration); it includes a component related to the urgency of treatment; and it must also – if it is to be practically useful for setting priorities – include an element related to the possibility of treating the disease (a very severe disease should not receive any priority if it is untreatable, and if care does not alter any aspect of its course). The severity of the disease thus turns out to be a very complicated and multifaceted concept, and thereby a rather problematic basis for a simple priority-setting system. Before we use it in priority setting we will either have to leave out some com-ponents of severity or find a way of balancing them against each other. Similarly, analyses of other key concepts in the priority-setting debate like social functioning or quality of life also show them to be very complex concepts which cannot be operationalized and measured in any simple way.

The Norwegian experience also showed that there were substantial practical problems in implementing the systems proposed during the first phase of the debates. In Norway a waiting list guarantee system had been implemented, based on the five severity categories of the 1987 report. It soon became evident that the system did not work in practice. Doctors were willing to game the system in order to gain advantages for their own patients. If a patient could get a better position in the priority scheme, many doctors were quite willing to reinterpret the 'severity' of the disease of the patient (Kristoffersen and Piene 1997). There were also several examples of the political decision makers caving in to public pressure, and giving treatments demanded by vocal pressure groups (e.g. IVF treatment) much higher priority than they should have had according to the rules of the system. In practice the system was thus undermined both from within and from without.

The Danish report of 1996 and the Norwegian report of 1997 both reach very sceptical conclusions concerning the possibility of devising compelling and rational priority-setting systems which can directly legitimize the priority decisions. At the same time they acknowledge the necessity to prioritize in health care, and they suggest that if we cannot find rule-based systems which can legitimize the decisions, we will instead have to devise priority-setting processes that can lend legitimacy to the outcome.

The Danish report argued that the minimal requirements for a democratic priority-setting process would be transparency and accountability. In the words of the Danish Council of Ethics:

> The Danish Council of Ethics is of the opinion that in planning the operation of the health service, and not least in connection with priority-setting in the health service, openness and dialogue concerning the decisions and concerning the background for the decisions made should be ensured. This openness is to be inward as well as outward. There should be an effort to ensure that decision-makers at different levels be aware – informed – of which priority-setting consequences different decisions entail. The issue is ensuring clearness, the necessary information being available, and that analyses have been executed of which consequences different decisions entail. At the

same time the public should also be ensured a higher level of information on which decisions are made at which levels, and which reasons there are for the individual decisions. Such openness is crucial to ensuring that individual decisions can be subjected to criticism and possibly changed on the basis of the public debate. For this reason great importance should also be attached to the health planning in the counties being organized in such a way as to ensure the possibility for common citizens to participate in the decision-making process, for instance at hearings and public meetings.

(Danish Council of Ethics 1996: 95)

It is important to note that the Danish and Norwegian reports do not claim that a good process is sufficient in itself to legitimize outcomes, and that a discussion of priority criteria and underlying values is therefore unnecessary. One of the inputs to the process will have to be some understanding of the societal values underlying the public health care system, but the claim is that even perfect knowledge about these values is not sufficient in itself to fix a given outcome. Both the reports contain extensive discussions about these values, and try to show how they might rule out certain kinds of priority criteria (e.g. priority according to social status). The Danish attempt at stating the goal of the health care system and the underlying values is as follows:

The furtherance of health and prevention of disease, fighting and relieving suffering related to health with the aim of ensuring the possibility for self-expression for all irrespective of social background and economic ability.

This goal should be seen in connection with a set of crucial values, which do not only apply to the health service, but to aspects of the welfare society as a whole:

Equal human worth
Solidarity
Safety and security
Freedom and self-determination.

(Danish Council of Ethics 1996: 93–4)

The Norwegian 1997 report goes much further than the Danish 1996 report in the concrete design of a priority-setting process which can legitimize priority decisions. The report recommends a fundamental revision of the system for setting priorities. Instead of a top-down system with one overarching definition of necessary treatment and care, a bottom-up system is recommended based on specialty-specific working groups. Each working group is given the task of explicating the specific meaning of the concepts of severity, utility and efficiency within its specialty. From these definitions the groups should move on to suggest a ranking of the various conditions treated within the specialty, and make recommendations concerning changes in priority. These recommendations are passed on to the political level which makes the actual priority decisions. It is recommended that this should be an ongoing process, and that the membership of the groups should be fairly broad.

In order to redress present inequalities in the system the report recommends that the first five working groups should be established for underfunded specialties:

- child psychiatry;
- adult psychiatry;
- medical rehabilitation;
- home care in the municipalities; and
- orthopaedic surgery.

It is further recommended that a more general priorities working group should be established with special responsibilities for stimulating public debate about priorities, and investigating public attitudes and ideas concerning priorities.

One of the effects of the implementation of this system would be that both the professional groups and the politicians and administrators would have to state their reasons for making allocation decisions in a very explicit way. As yet this new system has not been implemented, but if it is, it will be a radical experiment in transparent and accountable priority setting in health care. In such a system the final decision will still be made at the political level, and politicians will still be able to deviate from the advice they have been given, but they are much more likely to be asked to justify such deviations since the advice from the working groups will be public.

In many ways the Danish and the Norwegian reports contain very similar ideas about the importance of focusing on the process of setting priorities. The two groups worked independently, but the similarity may be due to the fact that the chairman of the Danish working group and the secretary of the Norwegian group are both sympathetic to contractarian approaches to priority setting of the type put forward by Norman Daniels and Thomas Scanlon.

CONCLUSION

The debate about priority setting in the Nordic countries has not ended. As is the case in many other countries, it is a debate which continues to emerge onto the public scene from time to time. New examples of individuals or groups who do not receive health care services that they want or to which they feel entitled continue to grab the public attention for a short time and generate debates about priorities in health care. Most of these short media-generated debates are, however, characterized by being fairly superficial. The conclusion is often that this unfortunate group of individuals should receive the treatment they desire, but the debate almost never includes a discussion of where the money to pay for these treatments should be found. Nordic politicians also still seem to have a fatal attraction towards making the shortening of waiting lists the most important goal of health care policy.

The recommendations in the most recent reports have not succeeded in changing the public debate overnight, from a concern with single issues to a more complex debate about structural and systemic issues. Such a change will take a long time to be completed.[3]

ACKNOWLEDGEMENTS

This chapter is a completely rewritten version of a paper previously published in the *British Medical Journal* (Holm 1998). It has been written as part of the research project 'EURO-priorities' sponsored by the European Commission, DG-XII research programme BIOMED II. The author thanks the Commission for its stimulus and support. All views expressed in this chapter are solely the responsibility of the author.

NOTES

1 As an aside I should probably mention that I don't think that supervaluation will help us here, or the introduction of new comparative concepts like 'on a par with' (Chang 1997). I believe that there are good arguments that these values are, at least in some practical contexts, truly incommensurable.
2 This criterion still seems to have a very strong attraction for politicians, and for doctors working in certain specialties.
3 Just as the final version of this paper was being written the Danish government reached agreement with the opposition parties on the

budget for 1999. In this agreement the opposition parties managed to insert a six-week waiting time guarantee for 'patients with life-threatening diseases'. No explanation was offered as to where the funding should come from, or what effects this would have on other parts of the health care system. This example illustrates both the strong political attraction of seemingly simple priority decisions, and the need for much more transparency in the process.

4

REACTIVATION OF THE PRIORITIZATION PROCESS IN FINNISH HEALTH CARE

Jorma Palo

Several countries have established a committee, working group or council for setting priorities, also called rationing, in health care. While it is generally accepted that the prioritization process is political, the politicians themselves are often reluctant to admit this and transfer the responsibility to physicians. Optimism is warranted, but easy and early solutions cannot be expected. The aspiration should be to move towards a situation where decisions pass the test of being reasonable in the sense of being publicly defensible and fair (Klein 1998). The process itself, whether it is fixed and technical or simply 'muddling through', will be slow and proceed only step by step.

Finland, situated between Sweden and Russia, is a country with a large land area of the approximate size of the UK but with only five million inhabitants. It has two official languages, Finnish and Swedish, but is otherwise culturally and racially homogeneous. It is a member of the European Union and has the world record in the number of Internet connections and mobile phones per population. It spends 7.7 per cent (in 1995) of the gross national product (GNP) on health care with 75 per cent coming from public and 25 per cent from private funds. A special feature is the almost total autonomy of the 450 local authorities or municipalities to spend funds raised through taxation. The country's central medical board was abolished 10 years ago so there is no centralized body to supervise the financing and production of local health care. Instead, there are several Acts and laws that are supposed to safeguard the delivery of health care services to all citizens.

According to the Act on the Status and Rights of the Patient that came into force in 1993, patients have the right to treatment according to need as determined by their state of health without discrimination but within the limits imposed by the available resources. The local authorities thus have very broad obligations, but the precise content of these is sometimes unclear. They can, for example, make decisions about allocations of examinations and treatments according to patients' status. This practice can lead to inequities based on where the patient lives, a development that would not be considered 'reasonable and fair'. The first signs of inequities in access are, however, already discernible.

ORIGINAL PROJECT

With these trends in mind the National Research and Development Centre for Welfare and Health (STAKES) initiated a project to look into prioritization in health care. As a first step it appointed a working group, set up on 1 March 1993, with the following tasks:

1 To identify problems related to the allocation of health care resources.
2 To develop principles that can be applied in making decisions concerning both service provision and individual entitlements.
3 To stimulate widespread public debate on how choices should be made, and the grounds and values on which these should be based.
4 To make proposals on how to maintain and evaluate decision-making procedures.
5 To participate in national and international debates about health care prioritization, research and development, and to compile and produce information on this topic.
6 To attend seminars dealing with choices in health care arranged by the Academy of Finland, the Finnish Medical Association Duodecim and STAKES.
7 To learn from similar projects in other countries and to maintain international contacts.

The present author was chairperson of the group and the nine members included three physicians, one nurse, one journalist, one theologian, one philosopher, one lawyer and one health economist. The group was assisted by three secretaries. It consulted a large number of experts on topics such as patient insurance, rehabilitation and perinatal care. A final report was published at the end of its working period (National Research and Development Centre for Welfare and Health (STAKES) 1995).

No directives were issued because the group had no executive powers. Instead, the report included a list of recommendations covering such basic concepts as health, health care, publicity, ethical principles, health benefit and duties of the state and local authorities. The starting point was agreement on the definition of health as the age-specific functional capacity of the individual.

The report and its recommendations were widely distributed but their impact remains unknown. Meanwhile the local health care authorities are under increasing pressure to reduce services, and several cuts have been made. Worried by this development the Finnish Medical Association Duodecim, a scientific organization that covers all medical specialties, decided to reactivate the prioritization process in which it had also participated in the early phase.

REACTIVATION

A small working group of six physicians representing the society, plus some University Hospitals and the Ministry of Social Affairs and Health, was founded under the chairmanship of Dr Risto Pelkonen, Finland's *archiater* (oldest among the doctors – an honorary title given usually to one physician at a time). A representative was also invited from the Finnish Association of Local and Regional Authorities, and a physician representing the young physicians' association was appointed as a secretary. The group began work in 1996.

A year later it was realized that an additional board with representatives from other interested parties was needed. The board, which was appointed by the society in 1997, consisted of 13 members representing STAKES, the Finnish Office of Health Technology Assessment (FinOHTA), the National Pension Institute, the Finnish Medical Association, the Finnish Association of Nurses, the Public Health Institute and some other organizations. While the working group holds a meeting once a month the board convenes only three to four times a year. The idea of inviting a representative from the media was discussed but rejected.

Several people have been consulted by the group, most notably

Ms Wendy Edgar from New Zealand who visited Finland in 1998. Members of the working group have also maintained contacts with corresponding foreign committees and have participated in international conferences on priority setting.

The present status of the reactivation process can be summarized as follows. The first step was the production of a summary report on the current situation. It began with a short description of the challenges facing the Finnish health care system and of prioritization processes adopted in other countries, described ongoing research and development in the field, and outlined detailed proposals for containing costs while maintaining the publicly funded system. The proposals were somewhat different from the recommendations published four years ago and were briefly as follows:

1 *Ethical principles:* proposal to found a permanent committee for setting priorities.
2 *Principles of examination and treatment:* national check on current clinical practices.
3 *Evidence-based medicine:* further official support for the Finnish Office of Health Technology Assessment.
4 *Continuous education:* both professionals and political decision makers should be involved.
5 *Cost containment and funding:* DRG-based services financed by tax money and insurance.
6 *Participation of the public and media:* open discussion with possible citizens' forums.

A large two-day conference, 'Prioritization – Choices in Health Care', with about 300 participants, most of them invited, was held in February 1999. A national expert panel, composed of 14 members representing local municipalities, patient organizations, business community, media and church, evaluated the summary report and made numerous changes to the future action plan.

The report now starts with proposals on how to promote health at national and local levels and lists the relevant ethical principles. The state government is responsible for a long-term plan to guarantee steady financing of the services. It also has a duty, in collaboration with local municipalities, to produce data on the incidence and prevalence of various diseases in the community. Evidence-based national and local examination and treatment programmes are then applied, together with continuous education and quality control. Information technology is used to create reliable statistics for the comparison of services in the various parts of the country and members of the public and the media are encouraged to discuss the prioritization process.

The panel rejected the idea of establishing a permanent committee for setting priorities. Instead, the current working group will continue its work, at least for the time being. Despite some critical voices heard at the conference and in the media, remarkable progress has been made since 1993 in the sense that the concept of prioritization is now unanimously regarded as an ethical (and not unethical) method of solving the conflict between perceived needs and the available resources. No 'Oregon-style' lists were proposed, but there remains the problem of what to do if the action plan fails to guarantee the same level of publicly funded services to everyone.

FUTURE PLANS

The organizers of the new priority-setting project hope that simply by increasing awareness of the need for prioritization some useful processes will be initiated, both at national and local levels. One current problem is opposition to, and refutation of, the whole concept. A major task will be to recruit politicians into priority-setting discussions and to educate them in health care ethics, health economics and other related topics. Good markers are also needed for follow-up since the usual international indicators, such as average length of life and health care costs as a proportion of GNP, cannot be used in national prioritization. This problem will be solved partly by developing the use of DRGs (Diagnosis-Related Groups), thus allowing reliable comparison of costs and prices between various regions and municipalities.

Monitoring these developments is especially important in Finland where local authorities are largely responsible for the provision of (publicly funded) health care services. This is the reason for the somewhat surprising proposal to strengthen the supervisory role of the Ministry of Social Affairs and Health. Some supervision can also be exerted by the newly founded National Board for Health Care Ethics, although it has no executive power. International collaboration is mandatory but founding a new National Institute for Clinical Excellence, as in the United Kingdom, is not considered necessary.

In spite of all these measures the gap between needs and resources may grow wider and ultimately lead to a situation where detailed prioritization lists must be considered. Meanwhile a great deal can be accomplished in understanding the organization and provision of services, an area traditionally ignored by both medical and social sciences. The future of the Nordic welfare state is nevertheless in jeopardy, a fact that should give strong motivation to all involved parties to set the right priorities for the right patients in the right places. A failure to do so could have catastrophic consequences. The present model may be one method to avoid that situation, which is the reason why we propose it as an alternative to solve – or at least postpone – more painful prioritization decisions.

ACKNOWLEDGEMENTS

I thank members of the working group, Mr J. Back, Dr M. Kekomäki, Dr J. Lindgren, Dr L. Niinistö, Dr R. Pelkonen, Dr M. Rissanen, Dr O.-P. Ryynänen and Dr J. Schugk, for excellent collaboration.

5

ISRAEL'S BASIC BASKET OF HEALTH SERVICES: THE IMPORTANCE OF BEING EXPLICITLY IMPLICIT

David Chinitz, Carmel Shalev, Boaz Lev, Noya Galai and Avi Israeli

Yours is not to complete the task,
Yet neither are you free to desist from it.

(Ethics of the Fathers, Chapter 2)

Israel's National Health Insurance Law (NHI), which came into effect on 1 January 1995, represents a major policy reform which has been described elsewhere (Chinitz and Israeli 1997; Shalev and Chinitz 1997). This chapter focuses on one aspect which, as in the case of health policy reforms elsewhere, has emerged as both central and problematic: namely, determining and updating the basket of services guaranteed to citizens under NHI. After some brief background on the Israeli reform, developments regarding the basic basket of services are described and analysed. We conclude that the Israeli case suggests a proposition somewhat different from that proposed by Mechanic at the last Conference on Priorities in Health Care. Mechanic argues that explicit rationing may have more of a role to play in decisions such as those concerned with the contents of medical care benefits packages, but less so when it comes to individual treatment decisions (Mechanic 1997). The Israeli case supports the notion that health reforms driven by both efficiency and equity concerns inevitably lead to a perceived need for explicit rationing which in the end is carried out implicitly, even at the macro level of decision making regarding entitlements under a National Health Insurance programme. It appears that the two types of rationing must coexist. The myth of explicit rationing lends legitimacy to rationing decisions made implicitly.

BACKGROUND: ISRAEL'S NATIONAL HEALTH INSURANCE FRAMEWORK

The National Health Insurance Law of 1995 was designed to build on long-standing features of the Israeli health system while correcting aspects perceived to be contrary to equity and efficiency. Until the introduction of the law, 96 per cent of the population of six million were insured by four non-profit sickness funds. Israel, with a high level of medical services and well endowed with medical manpower (more than three physicians per thousand population) was spending about 8.8 per cent of gross domestic product (GDP) on health (Bin Nun and Ben Ori 1997). Despite nearly universal coverage and favourable health input indicators, pressure for reform built up during the early 1990s due to increasing financial deficits of the largest of the four sickness funds, inequity due to selective enrolment by some of the funds, and growing private finance of health services (Shalev and Chinitz 1997).

Under NHI, all citizens are required by law to join one of four non-profit sickness funds which, unlike previously, must accept anyone who wishes to enrol. Citizens may switch sickness funds once a year, introducing an element of 'managed' competition. Sickness funds receive a risk-adjusted (based on age) capitation payment from the government which is to be used to provide a standard basic basket of services defined by law. The basket listed in the law is extremely comprehensive, covering preventive care, as well as almost all acute care in both the community and the hospital. There is no price competition among the funds over provision of the basic basket; sickness funds may charge extra premiums only for supplemental insurance which does not cover services included in the basic basket.

An interesting provision concerns financing the basic basket. The NHI law sets the cost of the basket together with an index for updating this amount each year. If revenues from earmarked health taxes are insufficient to cover this cost, the government is required to make up the difference. For reasons described at length elsewhere

(Chinitz 1995), despite this legislative attempt to guarantee adequate funding, the amount the government is required to provide from general tax revenues is a constant source of controversy. Partly as a result, the health system under NHI is suffering a large deficit. It should be noted that some argue that the increase of overall health expenditures to over 8 per cent of GDP in 1995 was due more to wage increases granted to medical personnel than to the introduction of NHI (Bin-Nun and Ben-Ori 1997). Nonetheless, financial pressure has made the question of updating the basket both more salient and more difficult. In particular, arguments rage over whether and by how much the budget should be adjusted each year, over and beyond general levels of inflation, to cover the addition of new medical technologies, as well as the growth and aging of the population. It should be noted that during the first part of the 1990s, Israel's population grew by nearly 750,000, or by more than 10 per cent, as a result of immigration from the former Soviet Union (Lissak 1995).

The law states that services may be removed from the basket only by approval of a parliamentary committee, and that new services may be added upon recommendation of the Minister of Health, subject to approval by the Minister of Finance and the cabinet. The NHI law authorized the Minister of Health to set up a committee of experts whose task was to specify the details of the basic basket in terms of waiting periods, geographical access and quality, and also established a multi-sector National Health Council charged with advising the government on health issues including changes in the basket of services and priorities. Finally, it is important to note that the law allowed for a transition period, originally three years and subsequently extended to an additional year, during which sickness funds could continue to impose conditions (e.g. cost sharing and other restrictions) regarding access to the basket of services which they had applied before NHI came into effect.

STAGNATING EXPLICITLY

The major result of these legislative provisions was almost total stagnation in the basket of services. Despite numerous requests to expand services, especially by the addition of new medications to the basket, by December 1997 only two drugs had been added. The inclusion of the latter in the basic basket was due to aggressive legal action taken by a group of persons suffering from multiple sclerosis seeking coverage of the new drugs under NHI. Ministry of Health attempts to attach administratively mandated clinical guidelines as conditions of access never withstood legal challenge. It seems that such guidelines can only supersede a physician's orders if they are explicitly included in the list of services attached to the NHI law (Shalev and Chinitz 1997). In the meantime, the special committee created to specify the details of the basket met infrequently, without major impact, and ultimately was dismantled as part of legislative activity described below. The National Health Council was equally ineffective.

During this period, sickness funds either kept strictly to the letter of the defined basic basket, or would offer services beyond the basket, apparently as part of competitive behaviour. For example, some of the funds offered coverage of the cocktail of drugs for AIDS, before it was explicitly included. However, at a later stage these funds withdrew coverage, creating confusion among the public and a groundswell of demand for inclusion of these services (Peled 1997).

EXPANDING IMPLICITLY

While the policy instruments defined by the NHI law failed to function, sickness fund deficits continued to grow, in part due to provision of services not included in the basic basket. Ministry of Finance budget officers attempted to fill the policy-making deficit by including major structural changes in the NHI law in the annual Economic Arrangements Bill which accompanies the annual state budget proposal. Passage of this bill is a condition for passage of the entire budget proposal; its defeat is tantamount to a vote of no confidence which causes the government to fall (Shalev and Chinitz 1997).

The Ministry of Finance explored several approaches to cutting or restructuring the basic basket as one way of reducing pressure on health budgets. A proposal to remove 'non-essential' services from the basic basket and transfer them to voluntary supplemental insurance was withdrawn under charges that this would create a two-tiered health system. The Ministry then suggested removing the detailed list of services from the law, leaving only general categories in the basic basket. Opponents of this idea claimed that it undermined the basic principle in the NHI law of consumer rights to a guaranteed basket of services. Finally, the 1998 Economic

Arrangements Bill included a proposal to allow the sickness funds 'flexibility' in determining their own service basket, subject to regulation by the Minister of Health (Knesset (Israel) 1997).

The Economic Arrangements Bill became the focus of intense public debate and activity on the part of interest groups. Coalitions of consumers' groups, specific disease groups, professional organizations and human rights organizations lobbied actively for defeat of the proposal to abolish the uniform basic basket (Shalev 1997). At the same time, a delegation of cancer patients, who had become concerned over access to cancer treatments, was received by President Ezer Weizman. In a nationally televised event, a young girl suffering from cancer pleaded to continue the treatments she was receiving (Cohen 1997). A few days later the government approved addition of 15 drugs to the basic basket, at an estimated cost of 150 million shekels, or about 1 per cent of the cost of the basic basket as budgeted under the NHI law (Peled and Greenstein 1997). The list of drugs to be added was based, in part, on the work of internal Ministry of Health committees relying on cost-effectiveness studies to develop priorities for adding services to the basic basket. Among drugs not included was one for treatment of osteoporosis as well as one for treatment of Alzheimer's Disease. The latter had been sought by families of patients with this disease and their protests received news coverage. Table 5.1 shows the drugs which were added and their anticipated cost.

In the wake of these developments, the Minister of Welfare demanded to be part of a ministerial committee on health affairs, together with the Ministers of Health and Finance. Following this, perhaps to compete with the rival political party of the Minister of Welfare, the Minister of Foreign Affairs similarly demanded to be included in such a committee. The very suggestion of such a committee of Ministers elicited cries of 'politicization'. Ultimately, the Minister of Foreign Affairs reversed his position and the idea of a ministerial committee was abandoned.

The final version of the Economic Arrangements Law allowed the sickness funds 'flexibility' in relation to the addition of services, while maintaining the current basic basket as a firm standard minimum. This basically copied the situation which had already existed. Since early January 1998, no more services have been added to the basic basket, though the government decided to add AIDS as one of several conditions receiving special reimbursement within the overall capitation payments to the sickness funds. However, 150 million shekels will also be allocated in the *coming* (1999) budgetary year

Table 5.1   Drugs added to basic basket of health services during 1998 budget process

Illness/function	Drug	Cost (Israeli shekels)
Platelet aggregation inhibitor	ABCIXMAB	10 million
Diabetes	Prendase	13 million
Cancer		100 million
Bone	Clodronate	
Breast, ovarian	Docetaxel, Taxol	
Various cancers	Epirubicine, Fludarabin, Gemcitabine	
Colon	Irinotecan	
Chemotherapy		
HIV/AIDS	Lamivudine, Ritonavir, Saquinavir, Stavudine	32 million
Schizophrenia	Olanzapine, Risperidone	
Total		**155 million**

Source: Memorandum from the Minister of Health to the Minister of Finance regarding addition of drugs to the basic basket of services, December 1997

for new services. A Ministry of Health committee made up of representatives of the sickness funds, relevant government ministries and public figures will deliberate on allocation of these resources. Whether the increment will become a permanent annual adjustment remains to be seen.

What did pass in legislation were proposals to permit sickness funds to levy additional charges, subject to approval of the parliamentary finance committee. Sickness funds have proposed, and ultimately received parliamentary approval to levy, new co-payments for medications as well as for visits to specialists and outpatient clinics. Proposals to allow sickness funds to levy an additional flat premium as proposed by the new legislation, did not, however, pass public and parliamentary muster. At the same time, sickness funds protesting budgetary constraints have taken measures to limit access by closing down clinics on Fridays, and to restrict choice of health care providers, for example by seeking to channel patients to their own, as opposed to hospital, outpatient clinics. These attempts are, perhaps, a form of implicit rationing, and have evoked some public protest reflected in media coverage. The new regime of co-payments has also evoked criticism. For example, for certain expensive drugs, sickness funds are allowed to levy co-payments amounting to 50 per cent of the retail cost. While co-payments for chronic patients are capped at 200 shekels per month, reimbursement for excessive sums is made retroactively to insured persons only once every six months. This causes cash flow problems for some patients, and entails subtle cost shifting when the insured fail to seek to recoup overpayments they have made, or cannot produce receipts.

In the meantime, the courts have continued to rule on suits related to the basic basket of services. In the case of *in vitro* fertilization (IVF), for example, insured couples have sued sickness funds which limited the number of treatments. In this case the court ruled that during the transition period of the NHI Law such limitations were legal. The ruling implies that after the transition period runs out, any new limitations must be explicitly specified in the basket of services with parliamentary approval. Incidentally, a national medical council on fertility treatments, a professional body appointed by the Minister of Health, has recommended, based in part on cost-effectiveness studies, limiting IVF to seven cycles for couples having two children or less. However, it remains to be seen how large a gap exists between the technocratic proposals of the committee and the political decision to convert the latter into law. It should be noted that recent public opinion surveys suggest that the Israeli public ranks IVF as a higher priority than mental health care, treatment of addictions and dental care, and ranks IVF much higher than did a sample of US respondents (Israeli *et al.* 1997).

CONCLUSION: EXPLICIT SUPPORTS IMPLICIT

The two main processes described above and the nearly three years of stagnation followed by intense debate which led to rapid and episodic expansion of the basic basket, seen pessimistically, reflect primarily the brutal realities of budgetary politics. Seen optimistically, as an example of the 'intelligence of democracy', the system has arrived at the conclusion that 150 million shekels should be an annual allotment for new services to be added to the basket. A Ministry of Health public committee will now suggest priorities for use of the funds. Services not included in any given round are not rejected 'explicitly'; they may have their day in another round of budgeting. On the other hand, services included will be done so explicitly, with clinical guidelines. The discussion of additions to the basket has thus once again become very explicit, but within a budget determined implicitly. The process received unprecedented media coverage, suggesting that the outcome was partly a result of public pressure. It remains to be seen how visible the work of the public committee will be and what, if any, will be the public reaction to its deliberations. While we are unaware of any studies regarding public reaction to the process described above, our own research suggests that, while the Israeli population places high priority on almost all health services, there is some willingness to consider limitations in the face of budgetary constraints (Israeli *et al.* 1997).

Needless to say, the situation is far from stable. Budget deficits in the health sector continue to grow, and pressures to add new services to the basket do not subside as the needs of a growing population and the continuing growth of medical technology stoke demand. There are obviously no simple answers. The question is whether the policy process concerning the basic basket described above represents a viable and accountable means of combining explicit professional methods of priority setting with the implicit 'muddling through' of political processes (Hunter 1995). The Israeli case suggests that explicit and implicit approaches to rationing and priority setting are not mutually exclusive alternatives, but rather complementary tools which support each other.

ACKNOWLEDGEMENTS

This chapter is an updated version of a paper presented at the Second International Conference on Priorities in Health Care, London, October 1998 and published in the *British Medical Journal* (Chinitz *et al.* 1998).

It benefited from interviews and discussions with Ministry of Health and Ministry of Finance officials, Members of Parliament, and consumer representatives, whose time and input are gratefully acknowledged. Responsibility rests with the authors.

6

SETTING PRIORITIES: 'AMERICAN STYLE'[1]

Carolyn M. Clancy and Marion Danis

The process of establishing priorities for health services 'American Style' is much like Americans themselves: dynamic, diverse and rarely drab. Financing of health care in the United States differs substantially from other developed nations: services are financed by an elaborate arrangement of private and public sources, and approximately one-sixth of the population has no insurance coverage whatsoever. Health care delivery is undergoing a profound restructuring as more Americans enrol in managed care organizations. Articulating and addressing health priorities thus represents the end result of a series of complex interactions between federal and state government policies; employers' decisions to insure or not, and how much coverage to offer; and clinicians' decisions – enriched by input from the media and the public. The urgent question confronting all nations – *who* gets *what* services, and *who* decides? – is particularly complicated in the USA because of the growing number of uninsured. The purpose of this paper is first to describe briefly the impact of historical influences and recent trends on the current character of priority setting in US health care, and second, to identify looming challenges and likely future directions.

HISTORICAL INFLUENCES

Tension between concern for individual rights and concern for general welfare has long been a dominant theme influencing the American view of government. This tension has shaped the structure of our government since its beginnings, as evidenced by the system of checks and balances deliberately designed by the founding fathers to limit government power over an individual's right to 'life, liberty, and the pursuit of happiness'. The federal government was further limited by shared responsibilities with the states and local governments. This circumspect view of government and the separation of powers has had a powerful impact on the role of the government in US health care (Churchill 1987).

Through incremental legislation over this century, the federal government has come to support many facets of health care as well as biomedical and health services research and the training of health professionals. In the absence of a consensus about the role of government in providing health care for all citizens, legislation has been passed to guarantee coverage for selected segments of the population considered deserving or in need: military personnel and veterans, the elderly (Medicare), and Native Americans; and partial support to employed individuals through a tax subsidy to their employers. Federal and state governments jointly fund the major programme for the poor and disabled (Medicaid). A safety net consisting of publicly funded hospitals and clinics complemented by unreimbursed care from private institutions has evolved to provide services for the uninsured. Overall, tax dollars pay for 43 per cent of all health care services.

While Americans have been reluctant to place responsibility for health care in the hands of government, they have had unbridled enthusiasm for the medical enterprise itself, as manifest by the unparalleled proportion of the GNP devoted to health care (Payer 1996). Until quite recently American physicians functioned as highly independent actors with almost unlimited discretion in clinical decisions. Priority setting has thus been as complex as the sources of financing, without centralized planning and budgeting.

RECENT DEVELOPMENTS

Over the last two decades, unremitting health cost inflation has stimulated discussion among private and public payers, though most attempted to address the problem independently. Fifteen years of unsuccessful efforts to contain costs and increased numbers of uninsured individuals culminated in a substantial failed effort to reform the entire US health care system in 1993–4. Subsequently, a default consensus favouring market-based solutions has emerged: health care 'reform' now refers to private sector innovations in health care delivery, with substantial discretion for priority setting delegated to negotiations between payers, providers and health plans.

An historic reliance on employer-based coverage is increasingly strained by a changing employment base. Losses in the heavily unionized manufacturing industries have been replaced by service industries which have been far less likely to provide insurance coverage for workers. Incremental, targeted efforts to expand coverage have not kept pace with the loss of jobs that include insurance benefits, so the number of uninsured continues to rise – both because not all employers offer coverage and because some low-income workers cannot afford the premiums (Cooper and Schone 1997; Bodenheimer and Sullivan 1998). Dramatic changes in the welfare programme in 1996, ending the entitlement that buffered the impact of economic changes, combined with widening gaps in the distribution of income, have increasingly strained the safety net as the multiple payers attempt to minimize cross-subsidies for the uninsured. A federal law that regulates pensions, the Employee Retirement Income Security Act, greatly limits states' power to raise funds to expand coverage for the uninsured (Copeland and Pierron 1998).

The majority of Americans who do have insurance are now enrolled in some kind of managed care organization, whose under-lying principle is the integration of financing and delivery of services. In recent years publicly-insured beneficiaries have also been encouraged (Medicare) or required (Medicaid) to enrol in these plans. Several states have developed specific plans to link enrolment of Medicaid beneficiaries in managed care arrangements with efforts to expand coverage for the uninsured by expanding Medicaid eligibility. Oregon used a very explicit process to incorporate public and expert judgements into a priority-setting process that ranked all possible medical treatments in order of appropriateness and importance according to 13 criteria. Though the process – 'rationing' – sparked considerable furore among politicians, ethicists, health professionals and the public, on balance the Oregon Health Plan has expanded benefits more than it has reduced them and has made coverage available to 100,000 previously uninsured persons (Bodenheimer 1997).

While the Oregon approach remains unique, rapid growth of managed care organizations, by definition responsible for providing services for a defined population, has begun to offer unprecedented potential for a population-based approach to priority setting. For the first time, large private employers and public purchasers have begun to work together to demand clear evidence of health plan performance (Bodenheimer and Sullivan 1998; Epstein 1998). Accreditation of health plans by a private sector organization, the National Committee on Quality Assurance (NCQA), now includes assessment of health plan performance in specific domains to inform purchasers and consumers, and is required by a majority of large employers as well as the Health Care Financing Organization (HCFA), the federal entity that administers the Medicare and Medicaid programmes (Iglehart 1996; Epstein 1998). NCQA's Committee on Performance Measurement brings together employ-

Table 6.1 Performance measures in Health Plan Data and Information Set (HEDIS) 99

Domain	Example
Effectiveness of care	Childhood immunization status Breast cancer screening Beta blocker treatment after MI Eye exams for people with diabetes
Access/availability of care	Children's access to primary care practitioners Initiation of prenatal care Availability of language interpretation services
Satisfaction with experience of care	Consumer Assessment of Health Plans Survey
Health plan stability	Disenrolment Practitioner turnover
Use of services	Well-child visits in the first 15 months of life Frequency of ongoing prenatal care Caesarean section and VBAC
Cost of care	Rate trends
Health plan descriptive information	Board certification/Residency completion Practitioner compensation

Source: National Committee on Quality Assurance, Washington, DC.
http://www. ncqa.org

ers, unions, health plans, consumers, providers and scientific experts to develop measures based on relevance, scientific soundness and feasibility. Performance measures are organized into seven domains and represent the first broad-scale consensus for standardizing how health plan performance is assessed.

Public reporting of performance in these domains is presumed to stimulate internal efforts at improving performance. Indeed, considerable resources are required to measure and then implement strategies to enhance performance in each domain. The active involvement of the Health Care Financing Administration with private employers in requiring health plans to demonstrate performance is an important component of a fundamental shift in a federal role – from acting as a passive payer to a 'value-based purchaser'. Selection of measures for assessment of plan performance has thus become an important component of priority setting.

Last, public concerns that managed care plans may have accrued too much discretion have diminished legislators' reservations about government regulation of clinical practice, and led to multiple bills that focus very specifically on one particular condition or practice, such as the 'drive-through' deliveries[2] and broader legislation for a Patient's Bill of Rights (Hellinger 1996b; President's Advisory Commission 1998).

In summary, the impact of these recent developments is that priority setting resides in the private sector amidst burgeoning efforts at public–private oversight. Delegation of authority to the private sector has changed the role of the federal and state governments as passive payers for health care to one of value-based purchasers, emulating and joining selected activities of large private employers. Thus the USA offers a picture of priority setting that lacks organization at the national level at the same time that it is likely to offer new insights about priority setting at the organizational level.

CURRENT CHALLENGES AND FUTURE DIRECTIONS

A number of specific challenges loom on the horizon and the US system is beginning to address them in characteristic fashion. We will focus on four challenges that we expect will confront all health care systems – changing demographics; advances in technology; economic instability and ethical dilemmas. For each we will illustrate emerging US responses.

Demographic shifts to a more elderly population with a high prevalence of chronic diseases – attributable in part to the very successes of medical treatments as well as universal coverage for the elderly – are a reality for all developed nations. Concerns in the USA focus on the future financial viability of the Medicare programme. In response, a bipartisan congressional commission on Medicare has been charged to rethink fundamentally the shape of the programme in the future.

Advances in medical technology exert persistent pressures on priority setting. Interventions that maintain function at high cost (e.g. organ transplantation with immunosuppression), interventions whose primary purpose is to enhance quality of life (e.g. Viagra), heroic but marginally or even questionably effective technologies (e.g. high-dose chemotherapy and bone marrow transplant), and emerging advances in genetic diagnosis and treatments all compete for limited resources. These advances set the stage for conflict between payers, patients and scientists, and pose a formidable barrier to all priority-setting efforts.

An example of a novel effort at setting priorities, linking coverage decisions with acquisition of scientific evidence of treatment effectiveness, is the response to a new surgical procedure for end-stage emphysema, lung-volume reduction surgery. Following a period of unrestricted access to this surgery, and a technology assessment that recommended a clinical trial, the HCFA asked the National Institutes of Health (NIH) and the Agency for Health Care Policy and Research (AHCPR) to co-sponsor a randomized controlled trial. While the trial is underway, Medicare patients can have the procedure reimbursed only if they are enrolled in the study. Whether this trial represents a new alliance between payers and the biomedical research enterprise remains to be seen.

At a broader level, the relationship between biomedical research investments and subsequent improvements in treatment has sparked considerable debate about how priorities should be set for publicly supported research. Disease-specific consumer organizations have been effective at multiple levels of government in advocating more research funding (e.g. women's health, HIV). Very recently, the Institute of Medicine published a report assessing the overall priority-setting process at the NIH, and recommended multiple strategies for increasing public input (Institute of Medicine 1998).

The predominant economic challenge is posed by the instability of world markets which makes predictions about available resources for health care tenuous. In the face of a currently growing economy and disappearing deficit, Congress enacted the Child Health Insurance Program, a federal–state programme to expand coverage for children (Rosenbaum *et al.* 1998). Any further efforts to diminish the number of uninsured through further incremental changes are likely to be affected by the overall health of the American and world economies (Aaron 1998).

Notable ethical dilemmas include privacy of personal health information; equitable resource allocation for disabled people and other vulnerable groups; and the impact of financial incentives on clinical decision making. The 'information age' now offers the potential to assess the relationship between stated priorities and actual clinical practice and outcomes in unprecedented ways, but the large databases required threaten patient confidentiality. In response, multiple bills have been introduced to protect privacy including one state law requiring patient consent for reviewing charts. Intense efforts are currently being made to develop a solution that protects privacy but does not make it prohibitively expensive for health systems leaders and clinicians to assess quality of care.

Broad interest among payers and policy makers in the value or benefit obtained from investments in health care delivery has stimulated the use of research methods to assess patients' preferences and values for treatments. The values obtained are a direct component of cost-effectiveness analysis and related techniques to inform resource allocation decisions. The question of whether and how the values of disabled and other vulnerable groups should be weighted to arrive at equitable priorities remains an ethical and empirical challenge (Power and Eisenberg 1998). The first prioritized list for the Oregon Health Plan coincided with passage of the Americans with Disabilities Act which prohibits discrimination against disabled people. Notably, subsequent review of Oregon's initial priority list with an eye toward concern for disabled people resulted in no changes in ranking for 85 per cent of the items (Bodenheimer 1997).

The new financial incentives for physicians to contain costs under managed care have created substantial public concern that physicians will be rewarded for providing too little care, and that physicians' financial interests will dominate patients' welfare. A small but growing proportion of US physicians simultaneously receive both capitation payments and a variable portion of their total payment 'at risk',[3] which creates an incentive to be parsimonious. This arrangement may obviate the need for managed care organizations to develop policies that explicitly establish priorities, but instead shifts priority setting to the individual physician or physician group. Since physicians contract with multiple plans that have diverse reimbursement strategies, the net impact is not well understood, but there is evidence that explicit decisions regarding use of selected new technologies have indeed been delegated to physicians (Steiner *et al.* 1997). While some safeguards are in place to minimize the impact of this conflict, there is little empirical basis to guide policies. Whether current accreditation and performance assessment efforts will be sufficient to counter public and professional misgivings about these incentives remains to be seen. Additional research on the impact of financial incentives and other strategies on managed care is currently in progress.

CONCLUSION

Responses to current challenges are as fragmented as our health care delivery system, and largely reactive. Our collective challenge is to learn from these multiple experiments as the basis for future improvements. We hope to develop the capacity within the health services and ethics research communities to study these experiments so that Americans can make informed choices about health care priorities in the next century.

NOTES

1 The opinions expressed here are those of the authors and do not represent official policy of the Agency for Health Care Policy and Research, the National Institutes of Health, or the Department of Health and Human Services.
2 The term 'drive-through' deliveries refers to a phenomenon in the USA where there was a substantial public outcry because health plans and insurers were encouraging increasingly shorter lengths of stay in hospital for childbirth (in many cases less than 24 hours). In the USA there is no universal system of postpartum home visitors, as in the UK. In response to this outcry, many states and then the federal government enacted legislation requiring health plans and insurers to allow women to stay in hospital for 48 hours after a normal vaginal delivery and 96 hours after a Caesarian section.
3 In payment 'at risk' the physician or physician group receives a total payment for clinical services provided and tests ordered. If the physician orders more tests, he or she effectively makes less money; if fewer tests are ordered, physician income increases.

PART III

PRIORITIES IN DEVELOPING COUNTRIES

7

HEALTH PRIORITY DILEMMAS IN DEVELOPING COUNTRIES

John H. Bryant

Consideration of priorities leads us to ask, Whose priorities? In whose interests? Linked to which policies? According to which criteria? To be decided by whom? Implemented by whom? At what cost? With what expected impact? This range of questions indicates that the reality of setting and pursuing priorities is not only a technical challenge, but has extensive social, cultural, economic and political parameters as well.

Here, we are taking the further step of including the concept of health priority dilemmas in developing countries. One might think, somewhat casually, that the basic process of selecting priorities, complex as it is, would itself be dilemmatic. Here we wish to give further meaning to the notion of dilemma, including that each of a series of competing options can be morally defensible; that different parties may have different views according to differing values; and that health, life and human well-being are at issue. Further, some of the most important health issues – such as determinants of illness or even the illness or disability itself – may in fact be largely unseen until revealed by research or sensitive experienced-based insights.

Formally, the planning and priority-setting approach begins with the identification of major health problems and determination of their magnitude in relation to various population groups to be served (Reinke 1988). Priorities are derived from assessment of the magnitude of the problems as well as the feasibility, including costs, and the likely impact of interventions, keeping in mind that resources are inevitably scarce in relation to needs. Specification of mission, goals, objectives, targets and standards provides a base on which differential allocation of resources can be based.

An example of a technically strong though complex methodology for assessing priority options is cost-effectiveness analysis, which examines cost differences among several potential programmes for achieving a specified outcome. The Johns Hopkins' studies of rural villages of Narangwal, India compared effectiveness and costs of three approaches to health care: nutrition + health care (NUTHC); nutrition alone (NUT); and health care only (HC) (Parker *et al.* 1983). They were able to demonstrate that comprehensive care (NUTHC) is most attractive in producing multiple benefits at little more than the minimum cost required to achieve a single benefit.

Another example, using a similar approach, was by the Aga Khan University in Pakistan, where the criteria of prevalence, seriousness, susceptibility to control and cost of control were used to weigh or score patterns of disease and hazards to health for priority setting. Application of those priority choices led to substantial reduction in infant and child mortality at modest costs in field sites of the squatter settlements of Karachi (Bryant *et al.* 1993).

However, while such methodologically based approaches, focused on defined local areas, can be beneficial, these examples as presented address a small part of the problems facing developing countries and global efforts to deal with major health problems. One challenge is that of going upscale so that locally defined advances are extended to larger populations. More generally, priority setting at country level in the developing world is fraught with uncertainty: health information may not be dependable; analytical methods for identifying priority options may not be in place; coherent processes for decision making may not be there; and obstacles to implementation may leave priorities as only hopes. At the global level, there is the problem of allocating resources across both the spectrum of problems and the range of countries with differential needs.

Our focus here is on developing countries, and it is important to note that priority setting in the more developed countries often takes on problems and methods that are somewhat removed from those usually addressed by developing countries. Chris Ham has laid out a detailed analysis of priority-setting experiences in a group of developed countries (Ham 1997). The priority decisions he discusses are focused mainly on matters related to patient care, and whether specific services should be covered by health services' financial arrangements or not. He concludes that there are no simple or technical solutions to the priority-setting dilemma. It involves a continuing process not amenable to once-and-for-all decisions. There is no right answer to the question, What should be our priorities? The answer involves a series of value judgements, which will vary according to the individuals and groups involved.

Two points are of special relevance to developing country processes. One has to do with establishing an explicit ethical framework or set of values, which is important not because it provides quick answers, but because such a framework helps to make clear the nature of the trade-offs that are involved. The other point has to do with public participation – techniques drawn from economics and other disciplines have to be used alongside debate if priority setting is to be seen as legitimate by citizens and other stakeholders. The lessons described by Ham will be increasingly relevant to developing countries that move toward public and private financing of health services with universal or widespread coverage.

Against that background of questions, uncertainty and experiences in developed countries, we will consider some perspectives that shape the context for decision making about priorities in developing countries.

EXAMPLES OF PRIORITY DILEMMAS

Here we will focus on five areas of challenge to illustrate the nature of priority dilemmas in developing countries. The first three examples provide opportunity for examining the variability in the nature and seriousness of the problems; the kinds of criteria for considering priorities; the sources of opinion or expertise for proposing such criteria; the location or level of impact of priority proposals; who makes the priority-setting decisions; and the chances for implementation. The fourth examines the place of research in helping to shape priority decisions at the policy level. The fifth moves beyond the boundaries of health priorities to the most serious threats to global well-being.

The five examples are:

- non-communicable diseases – moving to priority concern;
- ensuring the place of equity in health care reform;
- child mortality, primary health care and the roles of communities;
- setting research priorities – working against the *inequity clock*;
- nuclear armaments – a priority issue of unique dimensions.

Non-communicable diseases – moving to priority concern

The spectrum of disease in developing countries is changing from one of predominantly communicable diseases (CDs) to predominantly non-communicable diseases (NCDs), most notably cardiovascular disease (CVD), which is understood to include not only conditions of the heart but also hypertension and arterial circulation in general (Howson *et al.* 1998). By the mid-1990s, CVD had become the developing world's leading cause of death.

In the *Global Burden of Disease Study*, which reported the distribution of deaths by region for 1990, NCDs ranked first in most developing countries, in developed countries and worldwide (Murray and Lopez 1997). Moreover, CVD usually accounts for about half of all NCD deaths.

Against that background, we can examine the policy implications of the National Health Survey of Pakistan, carried out by the Pakistan Medical Research Council (Pakistan Medical Research Council 1997). This study, carefully executed and based on primary sampling units around the country, included both household interviews and physical examinations, including blood pressure and blood sugar determinations. Findings relating to hypertension included the following:

- The prevalence in adults ranged from 12 per cent to 33 per cent in the general population, varying with age, gender, body mass index and economic status. In persons 40 years of age and over, the prevalence ranged from 20 per cent to 65 per cent, being highest in obese, urban women.
- Of those found to be hypertensive, 60 per cent to 90 per cent (depending on rural or urban location) were unaware of it, and of those aware, only a small proportion were treated and under control.
- A similar pattern, though with lesser prevalence, was seen with diabetes.

It is fair to say that the population is not well informed about hypertension and other NCDs, nor about risk factors related to them and the steps that can be taken in support of health promotion, disease prevention and treatment. The data on hypertension can be viewed in the context of Pakistan as a developing country with closely limited resources, a health care system that is largely underfunded, understaffed and under-managed. Further, the double burden of communicable and non-communicable diseases must be acknowledged, so both can be included among priority concerns. Current efforts to develop national health policies are well formulated but with limited possibilities for early implementation.

Here is clear evidence for establishing hypertension and other NCDs as priority problems, but the resources and health system capacities for effective response are absent.

Ensuring the place of equity in health care reform

Equity is the centrepiece of WHO's health policy document – *Health for All in the 21st Century* (WHO 1997). The pursuit of equity calls for diminishing inequalities in health status. Another expression of equity acknowledges that different people and populations have differential needs, and equity calls for health care that is responsive to those differing needs.

It is one thing to design primary health care (PHC) systems that are equity-oriented, as we have done in selected sites in Pakistan (Bryant *et al.* 1993). A larger challenge is to pursue equity on a national basis through steps of health care reform. Given the complexity of emerging versions of health care reform, how is equity to be ensured? Norman Daniels and his colleagues have developed *Benchmarks of Fairness for Health Care Reform* (Daniels *et al.* 1996*)*, which can be used as a tool for assessing the fairness (or equity) inherent in reform options (see Table 7.1).

As examples of their applications, when applied to health care reform options then before the US Congress, a legislative proposal that followed the pattern of the single payer system of Canada scored very highly in terms of fairness, while one that was strongly market oriented achieved quite a low score.

Daniels and his colleagues, including ourselves, are in the process of adapting the benchmarks to developing country settings. This can provide a policy-related tool for assessing priority options in terms of equity. Such a tool could support constructive dialogue among interested parties in formulating equity-oriented health policies.

Child mortality, PHC and the roles of communities

Our experience with child mortality in the squatter settlements of Karachi brings some special lessons for priorities in health care. The Aga Khan University (AKU) developed a community-based, equity-oriented PHC programme that resulted in a decrease in the Infant Mortality Rate (IMR) from 126 to 60 over a period of five

Table 7.1   Benchmarks of fairness for health care reform

1   Universal access – coverage and participation
    Mandatory coverage and participation
    Prompt phase-in
    Full portability and continuity of coverage
2   Universal access – minimizing non-financial barriers
    Minimizing maldistribution of personnel, equipment, facilities
    Reform of health professional education
    Minimizing language, cultural, class barriers
    Minimizing educational and informational barriers
3   Comprehensive and uniform benefits
    Comprehensiveness: all effective and needed providers.
    No categorical exclusion of services, like mental health or long-term care
    Reduced tiering and uniform quality
    Benefits not dependent on savings
4   Equitable financing – community-rated contributions
    True community-related savings
    Minimum discrimination via cash payments
5   Equitable financing – by ability to pay
    All direct and indirect payments and out-of-pocket expenses scaled to household budget and ability to pay
6   Value for money – clinical efficacy
    Emphasis on primary care
    Emphasis on public health and prevention
    Systematic assessment of outcomes
    Minimizing over-utilization and underutilization
7   Value for money – financial efficiency
    Minimizing administrative overheads
    Tough contractual bargaining
    Minimize cost shifting
    Anti-fraud and abuse measures
8   Public accountability
    Explicit, public and detailed procedures for evaluating services
    Explicit democratic procedures for resource allocation
    Fair grievance procedures
    Adequate privacy protection
9   Comparability
    A health care budget so it can be compared to other programmes
10 Degree of consumer choice
    Choice of primary care provider
    Choice of specialists
    Choice of other health care providers
    Choice of procedure

Source: Daniels *et al.* 1996

years at a cost of about $4 per person in the population per year (D'Souza 1997).

However, curiously, it became apparent that the IMR had levelled out at about 60, raising the question of why it did not continue to diminish. After some inquiry, and discussions with the community, we began to understand that some households were resistant to change, and that risk factors affecting those households rendered them less responsive to the usual PHC approaches.

One of the AKU team, Dr Rennie D'Souza, focused on this set of problems by undertaking an analysis of risk factors for child mortality (D'Souza 1997). By identifying 222 households in those communities in which mortality in children occurred due to pneumonia or diarrhoea, and 419 households where children had those health problems but did not die, she was able to focus on factors associated with mortality. Matched analysis of the cases and their controls yielded a number of risk factors, including the following:

- Households where the mother was illiterate had a seven times greater likelihood of a child death than households where the mother had five years of education.
- Where the mother lacked cultural autonomy for child care decisions and actions (the husband and mother-in-law controlled those matters), there was a five times greater likelihood of a child death than where that autonomy was not lacking.
- Where a traditional healer was used for treating those conditions, there was a 15 times greater likelihood of child death.
- A working mother who left her child without adequate child care resulted in seven times greater likelihood of child death.

We had not been fully aware of these factors that limited the capacities of families to respond to the usual approaches of PHC. Once that awareness was raised, it became clear that the community itself was a necessary intermediary in helping the health team in relating to these households. It was the community that could effectively discuss matters such as maternal autonomy and what constitutes adequate child care, and promote appropriate responses by the community.

In short, here is an example in which those responsible for health care had not seen critical determinants of the disease burden, and when socially sensitive research approaches revealed those determinants, new avenues were opened for addressing health problems – actually new priorities – which led to new partnerships, as with communities.

Setting research priorities – working against the *inequity clock*

Policy makers must be aware of the dangers of creating policy without evidence or information. Research and development (R&D) can be a powerful tool, and used appropriately can help in the setting of priorities and making informed decisions.

The Commission on Health Research for Development (1990) evaluated the distribution of resources for health research and determined that 90 per cent of global health research resources were focused on patterns of disease that afflicted only 10 per cent of the population. Those losing the benefit from this disequilibrium are predominantly the poor and marginalized people of the developing world (Hyder 1999).

This situation raises questions of equity, need, justice and global power dynamics. Thus, at the beginning of this decade a call was issued to change that situation, leading to the promotion of the concept of Essential National Health Research and encouragement of developing countries to delineate their own research agendas.

The Ad Hoc Committee on Health Research Relating to Future Intervention Options was then established under the auspices of WHO (1996) with the intent of strengthening global capacities to provide the information required for better decisions for health system development. The committee's work was carried out in synergy with the *Global Burden of Disease* study and extended the work of the World Bank's *World Development Report* 1993 (Hyder 1999).

A problem of considerable importance has been the time lag between the development of useful scientific information and its availability for those most in need. The 'inequity clock', as it has been termed, reflects the vital delay in the benefit of health research reaching those who can benefit most, such as the poor of developing countries.

One of the central contributions of the Ad Hoc Committee has been the identification of specific areas where further investments in research would make a difference to global health. These were labelled 'best buys', based in part on an analytic process involving five questions (Hyder 1999):

- How large is the health problem (magnitude)?
- Why is it not being adequately dealt with (persistence)?
- How much do we know already (knowledge base)?
- Is the planned research likely to yield interventions significantly better than the existing ones (cost-effectiveness)?
- How much is being spent already (current status)?

The Ad Hoc Committee attempted to make the disequilibrium in global health R&D resource allocations more explicit and transparent. This led to a greater sensitization of researchers and policy makers to the importance of work in the priority areas. When combined with the whole body of knowledge that includes elements of the burden of disease, cost-effectiveness and prioritization methods, there has been a catalytic effect on attracting resources to some of the priority areas. There has been increased funding for work on malaria vaccine, global anti-microbial resistance, a vaccine for HIV/AIDS, and new contraceptives, with more expected to follow (Hyder 1999).

The Global Forum for Health Research, a newly established organization closely related to the work of the Ad Hoc Committee and WHO, is playing an important role in identifying and monitoring areas on the global health R&D priority list. Further development of both methods and tools for priority setting will follow, and revisions of such lists to keep pace with those developments will be necessary. Tracking progress in such priority areas may serve as an indicator for global commitment to R&D for health problems of the poor.

Here is the possibility of working against the inequity clock – of both providing research-based information that can undergird policies that are in support of equity and also diminishing the time lag for doing so.

Nuclear armaments – a priority issue of unique dimensions

India and Pakistan tested nuclear weapons in 1998, to the distress of much of the world. Their reasoning is complex, to be sure, including security concerns. The point here is not to examine the reasoning, nor analyse the impact on the social, economic and political development of South Asia and the world, but to point out two aspects of this distressing event. One has to do with its potential impact on local approaches to health care where resources are scarce at best, a scarcity now aggravated by the diversion of resources from health and other basic human needs toward already large defence budgets. In terms of considering priorities, decisions to deploy such weapons are impossibly beyond the reach and access of any of the actors whose voices are ordinarily heard in health-related priority setting and policy formulation.

The other aspect has to do with the fundamental global insecurity involved in the testing of nuclear weapons, which raises the question, What kind of priority should this problem have in the minds and actions of health personnel? Here is a brief review of some actions being taken by those who give this problem priority in their own professional actions.

A press conference in Chicago at the offices of the *Journal of the American Medical Association* on 4 August 1998 focused on an editorial statement from the Presidents of the Indian and Pakistani Medical Associations, together with Dr William Foege and Nobel Peace Laureates Dr Bernard Lown and Dr Yevgueni Chazov, appealing to the Prime Ministers of India and Pakistan for nuclear sanity, and for commitment to no first use of nuclear weapons (Lown *et al.* 1998). They say, in the aftermath of the testing of nuclear weapons by India and Pakistan,

> A nuclear conflict between India and Pakistan would be an unmitigated catastrophe, not only for the people of India and Pakistan, but for all humankind. The military policy of both superpowers during the cold war was to strike first in time of crisis. Pakistan and India, sharing a border, have inadequate time for crucial decision-making and, with human reaction time being too slow for hair-trigger readiness, these life and death judgements will increasingly be relegated to computer systems. Ultimately, the bomb takes command of a country's destiny. Nuclear war is an accident waiting to happen. An immediate powerful trust-building measure would be to pledge no first use of nuclear weapons.

This press conference was linked to two articles: in the *Journal of the American Medical Association* (Forrow and Sidel 1998), and in the *New England Journal of Medicine* (Forrow *et al.* 1998). These articles review the history and current status of progress and set-backs in efforts to contain uses of nuclear weapons, and the roles of physicians in that process, and represent candid, stark, insistent messages.

Where does this fit into the health priority dilemmas of developing countries? There are many in the health sector of those two nations, as well as of other developing nations, who are speaking out and taking action, trying to focus urgent attention and action on this immensely dangerous problem. Is this kind of problem to be seen as a distraction from pursuit of health care priorities? Or is it a prime example of the factors that render priority setting dilemmatic?

CONCLUSION

Considering priority dilemmas in developing countries provides an opportunity to view the intricate choices facing decision makers in those settings. Decision makers in all countries are faced with difficult and complex decisions, trying to balance health needs against resources, when the resources are inevitably scarce relative to need, even in the most prosperous of developed countries. Developing countries carry added burdens of underdevelopment that multiply the distances between needs and resources, and between methods required for confident decision making and the realities of local capabilities.

These challenges – the great gaps between human needs and response capacities – confront decision makers, whether local health personnel at district or community level, national policy makers or international organizations, with a range of choices, seen and unseen, that define the concept of dilemma: a puzzling array of options, in which the accessible alternatives fall far short of what is desired. Nonetheless, there are inspiring examples of analysis and response that illustrate how health personnel in developing countries can join hands with others, locally and internationally, to respond to these challenges to advance the well-being of their people and of human kind more generally.

ACKNOWLEDGEMENT

Appreciation is extended to Dr Adnan Hyder, consultant to the Global Forum for Health Research, for his helpful guidance in considering the area of research priorities.

8

PUBLIC HEALTH PRIORITIES AND THE SOCIAL DETERMINANTS OF ILL HEALTH

Kausar S. Khan

This chapter focuses on those countries with the worst health indicators and considers the relevance of conventional approaches to priority setting in health policy. It asks the reader to consider whether priority should continue to be given to efforts to change individual behaviour among vulnerable people, or whether instead it is more important to concentrate on changing the fundamental structures of society which determine human behaviour. It is argued that the level of 'disorganization' of a society is the major determinant of the health of the vulnerable. Achieving improvements depends, therefore, not on technical interventions alone but on building partnerships with vulnerable people so they can become agents of change in their own social context. This, it is argued, is a matter of human rights. Unless priority is given to building local capacities to address local problems, the health status of the poor will remain fragile and neglected, which could be considered a gross violation of human dignity and rights.

IMPORTANCE OF SOCIAL CONTEXT

First it is important to consider the relationship between health status and the 'organizational state' of a society. Consider the following three case studies:

Case 1: baby with Down's Syndrome

An elderly primigravida has delivered a 3 kg female child. This birth has occurred after several previous failed pregnancies. On initial examination the resident medical officer notes that the baby has features consistent with Down's Syndrome and the suspected condition, implications and prognosis are discussed with the parents. At day one the baby develops abdominal distension and bilious vomiting. Evaluation reveals that she has duodenal atresia, requiring surgical correction. The cardiovascular system is normal. The father absolutely refuses any surgery and demands to take the child home.[1]

Case 2: 17 widows, 35 orphans

In a remote district in Pakistan nine men living in the same village are killed because of tribal enmity. As a result, 17 women become widows, and 35 children become orphans.[2]

Case 3: malnutrition among rural children

In a desert region in Pakistan there is a village that is a little over one hour's drive in a four-wheel-drive vehicle from the nearest urban centre, which is also the district headquarters. Once a week, the Second World War truck that functions as a public bus comes to the village.

In this village, anthropometric measurements of 19 children under 3 years of age showed that eight children were normal for their age, six were moderately malnourished and five were severely malnourished. The mother of a severely malnourished six-week-old baby said: 'I have no milk in my breast, so what should I feed the baby? I tried giving powdered milk, but the child developed diarrhoea. Now I give the baby goat's milk. At least there is no diarrhoea, but the baby is still very weak. Twice I visited the doctor . . . yet there is no difference in the child.' With sunken cheeks and tired eyes, the child lay listless in her lap.[3]

Two questions can be raised about the case studies. What do these examples tell us about the health status of the vulnerable and the social status of women and children? What do they tell us about the relative importance of individual behaviour and social structures?

It is quite obvious that there is an inextricable link between the health status of children in the three cases above, the status of women, and the conditions prevailing in the society (availability of transport, and quality of service). If a typical case of maternal death were to be added to the three cases above, the link between women's health and their position in society would be more intensely apparent. Add to it an abjectly poor public transport system and poor quality of care, and the stark realities of the social context that strangulates the health of the physically and socially vulnerable become glaringly apparent. These realities, it must be noted, include not only the physical/biological *conditions* of the vulnerable, but also their *position* in society. The conceptual dyad of *condition-and-position* is related to their practical needs and highlights the importance of gender-sensitive analysis and planning, taking account of another conceptual dyad, *practical-and-strategic* needs:

> Practical needs are related to the condition of women and their present workload and responsibilities. They refer to, for example, the need for a clean and nearby water supply, stoves for more efficient cooking, credit schemes or seeds. These needs can be addressed by practical and short-term development interventions, but are in themselves unlikely to change unequal aspects of gender relations ... Strategic needs arise from the analysis of women's subordination to men, and are related to changing women's position. These needs may include equal access to decision-making power, getting rid of institutionalised discrimination in the areas of labour, land ownership, and education, measures to eradicate male violence against women, and shared responsibility with men for child rearing.
>
> (Williams *et al.* 1994)

In the context of women's health and the health of vulnerable groups in general, determining health priorities from the perspective of the two conceptual dyads mentioned above is linked to the type of analysis that is undertaken. Two approaches to analysis of a situation can be invoked.

Consider the following example: a thief is caught, and two positions are taken on the reason for his crime. The first interpretation says he is the 'bad' guy; there is something wrong with him, so the priority is to change his behaviour, in this case by punishing him.

The second analysis argues that society did not give him adequate opportunity to be gainfully employed, hence he took recourse to robbery. Thus, while he needs to be rehabilitated, the society also needs to change.[4] So the two types of analysis are as follows: (a) the individual is at fault, so his behaviour must change, or (b) the organization of society is the main determinant of human behaviour, so social change is essential. The first position can be called a *functional analysis* of a situation, while the second position represents a *structural analysis*.

Let us now look at the first three cases and consider the implications of functional and structural analysis of the cases (Table 8.1).

The importance of considering both functional and structural approaches to health problems has been argued by Lynn Freedman, a women's health advocate:

> ... my point is not to deny that health has biological dimensions or to belittle the importance of physical health as a worthwhile policy goal; rather, my point is to show that even an individual's physical health – not to mention her mental and emotional health – is inextricably tied to the wider conditions of her life. Thus, physical health cannot be detached from political and social concerns, posited as an objective state of biological being, and then treated as though the choices we make in pursuit of it are apolitical and compelled by some internal logic that derives solely from health itself.
>
> (Freedman 1995)

This helps to emphasize the point that if the goal is to improve the health of the vulnerable, it is not enough to focus on the quality of services. A focus on the wider public health system is essential. It is in the social context that long-term changes need to take place if the health of the poor and vulnerable is to be placed on a self-sustaining foundation. It is well known that mortality began to decline in many countries of the North long before vaccines and antibiotics became available. The social changes that laid the foundations of better health for all in many countries of the North, sometimes referred to as 'the spirit of 1844', did not occur in most countries of the South. Though the scope of this chapter does not permit further analysis of why this did not happen, it is worth noting that better health in the North is based on structural changes without which these countries could be in a predicament comparable to that of many countries of the South.

Table 8.1 Different analyses will highlight different concerns

CASES	Functional analysis (focus is on the individual)	Structural analysis (focus is on social structures)
Down's Syndrome	The father is the 'villain', sees the infant's death as being in her best interest, and says: 'She is a girl . . . what life would she have?'	• How social structures function – inclusive of economic, political and cultural practices. Other concerns would entail the state of the physical infrastructure (public transport, water and sanitation) and resource allocation; and who has access and control over what resources.
9 men killed; 17 women become widows; 35 children orphaned	Behavioural change needed in the men who were killed; and in the 17 women married to the 9 men	• The judicial system – what are the laws and how does the judiciary function? How much autonomy does the judiciary have? What is the role and accountability of the law-enforcing agencies?
Remote village – out of 19 children under three years of age 5 are severely malnourished; 6 moderately malnourished	Behavioural change needed in the women; in the doctors in remote urban centres; in the women's husbands	• Extent of human rights violations; level of maturity of human rights groups and women's groups. Is there a popular movement for human rights? Is there a women's movement?

THE PROBLEMS OF 'DISORGANIZED' COUNTRIES

There is nothing really mysterious about the differences between societies with very poor health indicators and those with better (or 'good') health indicators. What is perhaps mysterious is the persistence of inappropriate ways of dealing with health problems in countries of the South, where services have been developed without giving consideration to the social context in which they must operate. As a result they fail to meet their objectives. The training programme of traditional birth attendants in Pakistan is a good example. Thousands of traditional birth attendants were trained but maternal mortality rates remain high. Similarly, despite the steady increase in the numbers of physicians and hospitals in Pakistan, women living within the hospital catchment areas are still brought in dead (Jaffery and Korejo 1993).

To help understand the context in which the health status of vulnerable people appears to be immutable, a simple two-by-two table can be used to classify societies with 'good' and 'bad' health indicators according to their 'organizational' status, i.e. how well organized or disorganized they are:

	Good indicators	Bad indicators
Organized societies	A	B
Disorganized societies	C	D

As must be obvious, most countries of the South could be found in category D. The case of countries in category B could pose very interesting challenges, but these will not be considered here. The purpose of the four-fold classification is, first, to illustrate the point that the health status of the poor is linked to the social context; and second, to show that the state of the society will determine the way priorities are set. From this position two conclusions can be drawn.

Conclusion 1: Many countries are 'disorganized', that is, they are politically unstable and have power structures that favour the rich and powerful. They have inadequate social sector development (e.g. water, sanitation, transport, food safety, literacy, etc.). There are wide gender inequalities; the judicial system is unable to meet the demands of justice and fairness in most cases (it is said that only 1 per cent of the accused in Pakistan are found guilty); there are high levels of corruption by state functionaries and a high incidence of human rights violations.

Conclusion 2: Priority setting amidst high levels of disorganization is, at best, *ad hoc* rather than planned, and at worst unrealistic or merely aspirational since resources are sucked into sectors other than health (for example, debt servicing, militarization, and maintaining the privileges of the politically powerful). These countries tend to score badly on health indicators.

These conclusions do not require formal proof to establish their credibility. They are obvious because they are so pervasive in countries like Pakistan. The issue therefore is not how to prove the link between levels of disorganization and poor health status, but *how* to determine which strategies are likely to be effective in overcoming the problems. In order to address the latter need (i.e. how to determine which strategies are likely to be effective) it is imperative that there is agreement on the common social concerns which must be addressed on a priority basis (not unlike, for example, the consensus on immunization against the six most important communicable diseases which is a common concern of national and international agencies working for child health), and that there prevails a common language of discourse that would allow a meaningful analysis to plan actions and strategies for addressing the priority area of concern (not unlike, for example, the language of health advocates who combine the language of human rights and reproductive health). Without these two basic conditions (agreement on the priority area for social change and a common language of discourse), a dialogue for priority setting would not be possible.

In order to have a dialogue between all those concerned with the health of the vulnerable, whether they are working in individual health facilities or at national, regional or international levels of policy making, agreement must be reached on four key issues:

1 Health improvement is not only a matter of providing health services; it is heavily dependent on socio-economic and cultural factors.

2 Ignoring the socio-economic and cultural determinants of health can lead to the nemesis of any scientifically sound intervention for health.
3 Priorities for health intervention must take account of the local context.
4 Participatory methods should be adopted to ensure that the voice of the voiceless is heard in setting priorities.

The following brief overview of health achievements and failures in the twentieth century will illustrate the importance of these four key issues.

HEALTH GAINS IN THE TWENTIETH CENTURY

It can be said most unequivocally that the best of this century is reflected in the overall steady improvements in the health conditions and health indicators around the world (Table 8.2).

Table 8.2 Improvements in the health status of children in three regions of the South

Sub-Saharan Africa	Middle East and North Africa	South Asia
• Decline in under-5 mortality from 25% in 1960 to 18% in 1993 • Increase in life expectancy from 37 to 51 between 1950 and 1990 • In 1980s 20% of children were immunized; in 1990s, 50% were immunized • Between 1960 and 1990, girls' enrolment ratio with boys nearly doubled in the primary schools	• In 1960, child mortality was 25% and by 1993 it was down to 7% • Immunization rates doubled between 1980s and 1990s • Between 1970 and 1990, enrolment in primary schools doubled • Girls' enrolment leapt from 28% to 70%	• In 1960, one in four children under five years of age died; and in 1990s, one in eight died • From 1960 to 1990, girls' enrolment ratio in primary schools increased from 29 to 62% • Immunization coverage increased from 28% in 1980s to 85% in 1990s

Source: UNICEF 1996: 46, 49, 50

Similar or even better improvements are evident from the global statistics:

> Over the past 50 years and even over the past 20 considerable gains in health status have been achieved. Globally, life expectancy at birth has increased from 46 years in the 1950s to approximately 65 years in 1995, and the total number of young children dying has been restricted to approximately 12.5 million instead of a projected 17.5 million.
>
> (Sanders 1998)

Moreover, there have been many impressive advances in medical science and technology, for example the development of laser therapies, dialysis, respirators, and other life-supporting machines. Alongside these developments significant progress has also been made in the international policy agreements which directly or indirectly affect people's health, especially those more vulnerable. These instruments help guide and critique health policies and actions. Some of the international instruments worth mentioning include the UN Declaration of Human Rights; the WHO Charter and the Primary Health Care Declaration of 1978; the Helsinki Declaration of Ethical Guidelines for the Protection of Human Subjects; the work of the Council for International Organizations of Medical Sciences, wherein for over 12 years a dialogue has been conducted on the issues of health policy, ethics and human values (Bankowski *et al.* 1997); the six UN World Summits in the last decade of this century; the UN decade for women (1975–85); and the Edinburgh Declaration on Medical Education in 1993.

Despite these advances, however, it is not good news for all and a far cry from the WHO aspiration reflected in its call, 'Health for All'. Inequalities in mortality rates among certain age groups have widened significantly between rich and poor countries and infant mortality rates actually increased in the 1980s in a number of sub-Saharan African countries. Reversals in health status have also been seen in the newly independent states of Eastern Europe and there has been a resurgence of communicable diseases (Sanders 1998).

Thus, the issue in the health sector, locally and globally, is not only what advances have been made for treating diseases, or where the setbacks have occurred, but what has been done to create the conditions for better health. Moreover, as conditions for health improve in some but not all countries of the South, inequalities widen. This trend is exacerbated by the globalization of the economy and the dominance of neo-liberal economic policies in powerful international institutions such as the World Bank, the IMF and the Asian Development Bank. This concern is most sharply and simply articulated by David Werner:

> For the poorer half of humanity, the goal of Health for All seems more distant today than 20 years ago. There are more hungry children in the world now than ever before. According to UNICEF, malnutrition contributes to over half of the deaths of young children. This year more than 6 million children will die because they do not have enough to eat. This is not because of total food scarcity, but because of unequal – and unfair – distribution. This is because some people have far more than a fair share of what the earth provides, and others have far less. It is because the world's ruling class has chosen a model of development, whose goal is the economic growth of the already rich, regardless of the human and environmental costs . . . For those on the bottom, there is little doubt that *health is determined more by the fairness – or unfairness – of social structures than by medical or health services, per se.*
> (Werner 1998, original italics)

In the face of these grim realities a series of questions challenge us all, provided we are prepared to place equity at the centre of health goals:

- What is available, and to whom?
- What is accessible, and to whom?
- What is affordable, and to whom?
- What is effective and efficient, and for whom?

These questions are not new but they have not yet been adequately answered, especially in countries where the old ethos of care has been replaced by an ethos that is characterized by misplaced priorities, mismanagement of national resources and unstable socio-political conditions. South Asia epitomizes this scenario, but there are also other regions in the world to which this general description can be applied. These issues are becoming more pertinent in view of economic globalization and increasing military expenditures by poor countries with formidable health needs.

CONCLUSION

Good and bad practices are to be found around the world. These are the common concerns of researchers, service providers and those attempting to demonstrate what is feasible in health services and systems. However, these groups often work in isolation and do not learn from each other. There is a need to foster mutual support, to create a common discourse and to build alliances for creating self-sustaining conditions for better health. This fragmentation in health development is particularly apparent in countries with skewed priorities such as India and Pakistan and it reflects a grave disrespect for the poor and the vulnerable.

If the tables are to be turned and the needs of vulnerable people are to reach the top of the priority list, the process of change will have to start where they are to be found, i.e. in the villages and urban slums. It is here that the differentials in health conditions and health needs are most apparent. These people must play an active role in priority setting. To achieve this their powerlessness and disillusionment would need to be overcome, and their voices heard.

It is relatively easy to establish the theoretical need for participatory approaches to local priority setting, but the transition from the rhetoric of community participation to its practice is the biggest challenge that mankind has faced. It is easy to sign a declaration of intent, but making it happen is much more difficult. For example, the UN Declaration of Human Rights was signed by most of the world's countries yet human rights violations are still rampant. The discrepancy between theory and practice can be quite overwhelming, but the latter appears less demoralizing when actual examples of local participation can be seen. Fortunately, such examples are available, even if they have not yet become the guiding principles for national policies (Norton and Stephens 1995).

Finally, it can be said that achieving the goal of Health for All will depend on changes in the socio-political context and in changing the balance of priorities between promoting global markets and safeguarding human rights. For effective and efficient health care of all, especially those most vulnerable, the social context has to change and health services have to be made more accessible and affordable, effective and efficient. The social context includes three critical elements: *health*, *society* and *capacity*. Without building local capacity, not only to give good clinical care, but also to mobilize the poor so they too can become equal partners in health care, the social context is not likely to change. Without the contextual change, the goal of health for all will be as elusive as universal human rights, and would remain a perennial struggle and at best only a fleeting reality.

NOTES

1 Case used in a short course on neonatal care, organized by the Department of Pediatrics, Aga Khan University, Karachi, September 1998.
2 Incident reported to the author by a participant in a training workshop.
3 Situation noted in one of seven rural districts in Sindh province, Pakistan, where the author coordinates a school nutrition programme.
4 One of the Khalifas of the early Muslim period is known to have suspended all punishments for robbery during a period of drought in his region. His argument was that he, as the custodian of his people, was responsible for food, and if this responsibility was not being fulfilled because of the drought, people could not be held responsible for theft of food. The emphasis here is on society's responsibility rather than on the behaviour of the individual, irrespective of the conditions in which he or she lives. In the context of health, this approach would mean that as the primary provider for the household, a woman is not solely responsible for the condition of her own and her children's health; the society and its norms are also responsible.

PART IV

ETHICAL DILEMMAS

9

ACCOUNTABILITY FOR REASONABLENESS IN PRIVATE AND PUBLIC HEALTH INSURANCE

Norman Daniels

LIMITING ACCESS BY DIRECT AND INDIRECT MEANS

Suspicion, distrust, and even resistance often greet efforts to set limits on access to medical services. This reaction rises to the level of a challenge to the legitimacy or moral authority of decision makers in the market-driven private sector of the insurance system in the United States. In some highly publicized cases, a similar challenge has been raised to the moral authority of decision makers in the publicly managed or regulated national health services or national health insurance systems. Providing accountability for reasonableness is key to meeting this legitimacy problem.

In the United States, private, generally for-profit employers and health plans set limits to care that have the potential to affect the health and welfare of those enrolled with them in fundamental ways. Some of these decisions are 'direct' ways of limiting access to services, such as coverage decisions for new technologies, decisions about the contents and design of a formulary, or decisions to limit access to specialists or certain categories of care. Other decisions 'indirectly' limit access by implementing novel forms of risk-sharing incentives with physician groups. These incentives, like fundholding arrangements in the British National Health Service, induce physicians to limit access to care and make them responsible for resource allocation decisions.

In theory, setting limits in the appropriate ways can improve the quality of outcomes of a covered population by eliminating unnecessary care, by implementing outcomes-based clinical guidelines, by assuring improved continuity and integration of care, and by setting fair priorities under resource constraints. In practice, however, limit setting is greeted with suspicion and distrust. Many fear that it is only the cost to powerful stakeholders in the private sector that drives decisions, not a commitment to meeting health needs fairly in a covered population. As a result, an increasing number of Americans fear that a treatment they need will not be covered by their insurer (Kaiser Family Foundation 1997), and they show increasing distrust of incentives to physicians (Kao *et al*. 1998).

Public suspicion about limit setting is not restricted to the United States, with its large market-driven private sector. Similar scepticism has greeted limit-setting decisions, especially where life-saving treatments are at issue, in countries with national health services and national health insurance systems (Ham and Pickard 1998; Edgar 1999). Public bureaucrats, like private managers, have been charged with making budget-driven decisions that are unfair or unreasonable. They are seen as paying inadequate attention to the needs or individual characteristics of individual patients and too much attention to worries about precedents and policy. In both public and private systems, there is an implicit challenge to the legitimate moral authority of those setting limits to make such decisions.

In what follows, I shall argue that we cannot assure the fairness or legitimacy of direct or indirect limit setting unless we implement forms of public accountability not now in place (Daniels and Sabin 1997). Specifically, we must go beyond demanding *market accountability*, the simple demand for clear information about options and performance that we hear in the United States, and we must instead implement measures that establish *accountability for reasonableness* (Daniels and Sabin 1998a). Accountability for reasonableness demands public access to rationales for limit-setting decisions. It also requires that these rationales be accepted by 'fair minded' people as relevant to meeting population health needs fairly under resource constraints.

Accountability for reasonableness requires a transformation of the corporate culture in which these decisions are made in the United States, for rationales for decisions would no longer be seen as 'proprietary information'. It also requires transformation of the bureaucratic culture that often exists in publicly managed systems, where, despite official forms of accountability to the public, it is often believed that keeping decisions made by experts 'close to the chest' is the best way to manage painful restrictions. In what follows, I shall illustrate how accountability for reasonableness can be established in key areas of direct and indirect limit setting in the United States, but the implications of these examples for public systems should be clear.

LEGITIMACY AND ACCOUNTABILITY FOR REASONABLENESS

Why should moral authority for such important and morally controversial decisions be lodged within private insurance schemes in the United States? Under what conditions, if any, should we come to view the exercise of such authority as legitimate and fair? (Daniels and Sabin 1997, 1998a)

A standard reply to this question in the United States is that when consumers exercise informed choices about their insurance options, then their choice of plan counts as 'informed consent' to the limits it imposes. According to this view, consumers need not know why plans set the limits they do, any more than they need know why car or computer manufacturers make the design decisions they make. It is sufficient that the limits are clear so that clear choices can be made. Questions about legitimacy are dissolved by the consent involved in the purchase of a plan – or car or computer – at a given price.

The fact that legitimacy requires consent and consent comes through actual *informed choice* shows the key limits of this view. First, nearly half of American workers have no choice of plans: their employers choose for them. In addition, many of us become aware of what limits mean for us only in the context of treatment, when it is too late to make another choice of health plan. Second, the enormous uncertainty that surrounds health care is different from that involved in the purchase of other goods (Arrow 1963b). We have better information about what our computer or automobile 'needs' are and how to match them to appropriate computers or cars than we do about our health needs and how to match them to appropriate plans, clinicians, or treatments. (This information problem makes our ongoing, interactive relationship with clinicians we can trust crucial to health care delivery but not car buying.) In addition, if we buy a car or computer that no longer meets our needs, we can sell it and buy one that does, perhaps with some inconvenience and cost, but without serious impact on our well-being. When a plan turns out not to meet our newly discovered health care needs, we may not be welcome in another one, or we may be too seriously ill to shop around.

Perhaps most important of all, if the computer market fails to provide us with machines that meet all our information managing needs, that is too bad, but no injustice is done. But if health plans fail to meet our needs fairly under necessary resource constraints, we violate a societal obligation to provide appropriate care for those needs (Daniels 1985), albeit a societal obligation that we have not adequately acknowledged in the political decisions I noted earlier. That means an injustice is done. There is simply no way to hold plans accountable for their role in meeting that societal obligation if we do not insist on accountability for making reasonable decisions. There is simply no way to guarantee that even an ideal market will provide people with reasonable coverage and treatment options without holding players in that market explicitly accountable for reasonableness.

To implement accountability for reasonableness, four conditions must be met (they are necessary but probably not sufficient conditions; Daniels and Sabin 1997).

1 *Publicity*: decisions regarding coverage for new technologies (and other limit-setting decisions) and their rationales must be publicly accessible.
2 *Reasonableness*: the rationales for coverage decisions should aim to provide a *reasonable* construal of how the organization should provide 'value for money' in meeting the varied health needs of a defined population under reasonable resource constraints. Specifically, a construal will be 'reasonable' if it appeals to reasons and principles that are accepted as relevant by people who are disposed to finding terms of co-operation that are mutually justifiable.
3 *Appeals*: there is a mechanism for challenge and dispute resolution regarding limit-setting decisions, including the opportunity for revising decisions in light of further evidence or arguments.
4 *Enforcement*: there is either voluntary or public regulation of the process to ensure that conditions 1–3 are met.

Condition 1 requires openness or publicity, that is, transparency with regard to reasons for decisions. If it is implemented, for example in decisions about coverage for new technologies or in decisions about the design of a formulary, then a kind of 'case law' is established. Plans reveal their commitment to appropriate reasons for limiting care through the demand that these constitute a coherent, defensible body of decisions over time.

Condition 2 requires the most explanation since it involves some constraints on the kinds of reasons that can play a role in the rationale. At its core, it recognizes the fundamental interest all parties in a co-operative scheme for delivering health care have in finding a justification they can all accept as reasonable. We can think of Condition 2 as requiring that we limit ourselves to reasons that 'fair-minded' people can agree are relevant to pursuing appropriate patient care under necessary resource constraints.

'Fair-minded' people are those who seek terms of co-operation that are mutually justifiable. In sports, we consider people fair-minded if they play by rules of the game that all accept. Indeed, fair-minded people want the rules of the game to promote its essential skills and the excitement their use produces. For example, they want rules that permit blocking in football, but not clipping or grabbing face masks, because they want to encourage teamwork and skill and not the mere advantage that comes from imposing injuries. Of course, having rules of a game that fair-minded people accept does not eliminate all controversy about their application, but it does narrow the scope of controversy and methods for adjudicating them.

Similarly, if the 'game' is delivering health care, whether in public or private insurance schemes, then fair-minded people will seek reasons they can all accept as relevant to meeting people's needs fairly under resource constraints. As in football, the rules shape a conception of the common good that is the goal of co-operation (or competition). In both games, people who seek 'mere advantage' by ignoring the rules, or by seeking rules that advantage only them, are not fair-minded. There will still be disagreement about how to apply the rules, but seeking mutually acceptable rules, as fair-minded people do, narrows the scope of disagreement and the grounds on which disputes can be adjudicated.

Conditions 3 and 4 provide mechanisms for connecting deliberation and decisions within Managed Care Organisations (MCOs) to a broader deliberative process, that is, for making them accountable to the results of a wider deliberation about what fairness requires in health care. The kind of appeals process required by Condition 3, for example, establishes a form of due process and helps open discussion about contested decisions to broader scrutiny. At the same time, if properly designed, these appeals should diminish adversarial confrontation in the courts (Daniels and Sabin 1998b). Condition 4 recognizes that public regulation may be necessary if self-regulation proves inadequate, but the combined intention behind the four conditions is to focus regulation on process, rather than on 'organ by organ' mandates in health plans. Current reform efforts contain elements of accountability for reasonableness, but they have not focused clearly on that as a central goal (Daniels and Sabin 1998a).

The guiding idea behind these conditions is to convert private MCO solutions to problems of limit setting into part of a larger public deliberation about a major, unsolved public policy problem. If the United States had a publicly financed health care system, as in Canada, Great Britain and many European countries, we might think that the way to address this problem is to do what the Netherlands, Norway, Denmark and Sweden have done, namely, form public commissions to frame general principles to be followed in setting priorities among health needs and services. There is good reason to believe, however, that general principles of distributive justice and general characterizations of the goals of medicine (Daniels 1996) cannot really address the problems of setting priorities in ways that satisfy our moral concerns in particular cases. Rather, we must seek agreement on how to make the practical decisions about limits that arise at various levels within both purely public and mixed public and private delivery systems. This point has been recognized in a second wave of commissions, for example in Denmark, that has focused on assuring a fair, transparent process of decision making rather than articulation of general principles.

In designing its rationing scheme for Medicaid, Oregon had to face this problem of reconciling general approaches with the difficulties involved in particular decisions. It developed a public process, but it had to revise its methodology several times, shifting, for example, away from cost-effectiveness rankings, to rankings by categories of benefits, to much more subtle adjustments and deliberations about their appropriateness. It is quite unclear whether any general principles really characterize the process or outcomes that resulted in the Oregon procedure. In many cases, the process ended up with commissioners making fairly specific choices in response to arguments and evidence about the rankings of particular services.

Since the US health care system is a mixed public and private one, key decisions will be made by private institutions that reimburse and organize the delivery of services for specific groups of patients. The four conditions we describe convert those otherwise private and localized decisions into part of a larger public deliberation about acceptable solutions to these problems of setting limits. There are reasons to believe that keeping the focus of problem solving within delivery systems may yield more coherent and defensible practices in the end than proclamations by public commissions – provided that these delivery systems are properly connected to a broader public deliberation and that the results of that broader public deliberation can modify or constrain the decisions made within particular elements of the delivery system. If met, these conditions help these private institutions to enable or empower a more focused public deliberation that involves broader democratic institutions. They may indeed be a model for how solutions should be approached even in public systems as well. The broader public deliberation we envision here is not necessarily an organized democratic procedure, though it could include the deliberation underlying public regulation of the health care system. Rather, it may take place in various forms in an array of institutions, spilling over into legislative politics only under some circumstances.

For private health care institutions to acquire legitimacy for their limit-setting decisions they must see themselves, and be seen by others, as contributors to a broader deliberative process that they constructively embrace. The four conditions that establish accountability for reasonableness contribute to a solution to the legitimacy and fairness problems by placing MCOs visibly in that role. Embracing these conditions and the way in which they connect internal decisions to broader, public deliberation clearly carries many of these organizations beyond the dominant perceptions they have of their organizational and (in many cases) 'corporate' culture, for it makes them accountable to more than their own boards of directors and in more ways than they are accountable to stockholders (if they have them). In an intensely competitive environment, embracing these conditions may be easier for associations of organizations than for individual MCOs, though it may also be possible to show there is some market value to having a visible record of commitment to patient-oriented decision making. If they are not embraced voluntarily and through self-regulation, then public regulation should require them.

ACCOUNTABILITY FOR REASONABLENESS IN THREE CONTEXTS

New technologies

Despite pressures to reduce costs, new technologies enter our health care system at a high rate and are viewed by many econo-mists as the primary force driving the rate of health care cost increases (Newhouse 1992). A three-year study of selected MCOs suggests that, despite intense competition and pressures to reduce costs, the evaluation of new technologies is done on a case-by-case basis, without the imposition of a 'budget' for new services that would force comparative judgements about their relative import-ance in meeting population health needs (Daniels and Sabin 1997, 1998a). There was little explicit discussion of costs or demand for, or use of, cost-effectiveness analysis in evaluating new technologies (outside formularies). Contrary to public suspicions, however, there is generally a very high level of deliberation about the evi-dence regarding safety and efficacy, and considerable attention is paid to designing 'mini-guidelines' to manage introduction of these technologies and assure reasonable quality.

What is missing, despite this high level of deliberation (in the select MCOs studied), is public accessibility to the rationales for decisions. Often, for example, a coverage decision for a new tech-nology is announced in a medical director's newsletter, and it speci-fies the terms and limits of coverage, including patient selection criteria, but it does not elaborate on the reasons and rationale for the limits to coverage. For example, when one MCO decided to cover growth hormone treatment for children who were growth hormone deficient or who suffered from Turner's syndrome, it announced its coverage limitation without providing a rationale for these limits. Adequate, reasonable rationales were discussed in the meetings of the coverage committee. These focused both on the limited evidence of safety and efficacy for an expanded population of very short patients, but also on the idea that uses of services for 'enhancement' of otherwise normal traits was not the mission of a health plan, whereas treating disease or disability was.

One problem with not being explicit about the grounds for the limits introduced is that an opportunity is missed to undertake both internal and external education about appropriate reasons for coverage (Sabin and Daniels 1998). If silence about rationales ends up implying that the coverage limit was based on limited evidence about safety and efficacy, then new evidence might reopen the coverage decision. If the plan had been explicit about invoking a resource allocation principle that gave priority to treatments over enhancements, then even if this principle proved controversial in some cases, it could be evaluated to see if fair-minded people considered it a reasonable basis for limiting care.

Health plans studied were fearful about transparency but were responsive to discussions about its importance. When the same MCO recently approved coverage for pallidotomy, a neurosurgical procedure for relieving certain symptoms of advanced Parkinson's Disease, it adopted the patient selection criteria used in the existing published studies. When it was pointed out that it was unclear whether these criteria arbitrarily limited access of patients who might benefit, the plan revised its announcement of its coverage policy to make it explicit about the grounds for the selection criteria. This plan had been persuaded that internal clarity about rationales would not only improve its own decision making, making it more likely it would arrive at defensible, coherent decisions across cases, but also that patients and clinicians would in time come to see that the pattern of reasoning underlying these cases was driven by reasonable concerns about patient welfare.

We have proposed generalizing these small steps to assure accountability for reasonableness by embodying them in National Committee for Quality Assurance (NCQA) standards regulating technology coverage decisions in accredited health plans. For example, Box 9.1 shows what a revised standard for technology assessment would look like if it incorporated accountability for reasonableness (proposed revisions are in italics).

There is room for this revision because NCQA already embodies concerns about accountability for reasonableness in some of its standards. For example, in providing an explanation (on its website) of its utilization management (UM) standards, NCQA captures their overall spirit with these questions. 'Does the plan use a reasonable and consistent process when deciding what health services are appropriate for individuals' needs? When the plan denies payment for services, does it respond to member and physician appeals?' In its rationale for the standard (UM1) that requires clearly defined utilization management structures, procedures and responsibilities, NCQA says, 'A well-functioning UM program manages the use of limited resources to maximize the effectiveness of the care provided to the member. By defining how utilization decisions are made, a well-structured UM program promotes fair and consistent UM decision making.'

Box 9.1   Proposed revisions to NCQA utilization management standards

Standard UM 7: The managed care organization evaluates the inclusion of new medical technologies and the new application of existing technologies in the benefit package. This includes medical procedures, drugs and devices.

UM 7.1: The managed care organization has a *publicly available* written description of the process used to determine whether medical technologies and new uses of existing technologies will be included in the benefit package.

UM 7.1.1: The written description includes the decision variables that the managed care organization uses to decide whether new medical technologies and the new application of existing technologies will be included in the benefit package.

UM 7.1.1.1: Allowable decision variables are restricted to those that appeal to evidence, reasons and principles considered relevant to the meeting of patient needs under reasonable resource constraints.

UM 7.1.2: The process includes a review of information from appropriate government regulatory bodies as well as published scientific evidence.

UM 7.1.3: Appropriate professionals participate in the process to decide whether to include new medical technologies and new uses of existing technologies in the benefit package.

UM 7.2: The managed care organization implements this process to assess new technologies and new applications of existing technologies.

UM 7.2.1: The implementation includes making each decision reached and the underlying rationale for it (including, for example, the rationale for patient selection criteria) publicly available in writing, thereby accumulating a 'case law' record of the reasoning employed by the organization.

UM 7.2.2: The implementation allows for new arguments and input from appeals so that decisions can be revisited in light of relevant information.

Quite correctly, NCQA recognizes that fairness and consistency must not only be present, but demonstrable to members. In its rationale for the standard (UM2) that requires publicly available utilization review decision criteria based on sound clinical evidence, NCQA says:

> The managed care organization must be able to demonstrate to members and practitioners that UM decisions are made in a fair, impartial, and consistent manner that serves the best interests of the members. Therefore, the managed care organization has objective, measurable UM decision-making criteria that are based on reasonable medical evidence.

Specifically, decisions must be consistent with clinical practice guidelines where they have been introduced, and they must be available and understandable to clinicians. At the same time, such guidelines cannot be viewed as 'absolute' criteria and must allow for variation among patients (UM 5). Here too, fair-minded persons would agree to the limits imposed by clinical guidelines only if allowance was made for the specific features of individual cases.

The rationale for the NCQA standard that concerns appeals procedures (UM 6) explains that 'accountability' for its decisions means an MCO that denies coverage must

> clearly explain the reasons for the denial to the member if the member was involved in the UM process, as well as to the practitioner, as appropriate. *The inclusion of the reason for a denial allows the member and/or practitioner to understand the reasoning behind the managed care organization's decision'* (italics added).

In sum, the member (and practitioner) affected by a denial of coverage is directly owed accountability for a full explanation of the rationale for the decision.

The most controversial technology coverage decisions health plans make are those that involve 'last-chance' therapies for fatal or severely debilitating illnesses. In these cases, there is considerable room for disagreement about how to weigh the values of stewardship of scarce resources and the generation of knowledge about effective treatments, which would incline plans not to cover unproven therapies, against the value of meeting urgent needs, which might lead to more liberal coverage of last-chance therapies. This moral controversy makes this a highly contentious area, and it is not surprising that a mechanism for external review of appeals has emerged as one model for providing due process in these cases. Accountability for reasonableness can be embodied in various strategies for addressing the disagreements these types of decisions involve, but I refrain from further comment on some of these 'best practices' here (Daniels and Sabin 1998b).

Formulary management

A small number of pharmacy benefit management (PBM) 'carve-out' companies now design and manage the formularies for half of all people with insurance. The two largest of them each manage benefits for over 50 million lives. The attraction of these companies is that they have been able to use their purchasing leverage to arrange discounts from drugstore chains and rebates from manu-facturers, slowing the rate of cost increase in formularies. In recent years, however, discounting has not been able to slow the rapid increase in formulary costs, which have risen far more rapidly than health care costs generally. Since a flood of new pharmaceuticals is in the pipeline of research and development, cost pressures will only increase. Indeed, Viagra brought to public consciousness the degree to which costs, if not cost-effectiveness, will play an explicit role in coverage decisions and plan design.

Formulary design involves decisions at several levels. First, there are 'categorical' decisions concerning the general types of pharma-ceuticals covered. A further 'drug selection' decision is then often made to cover only some drugs within the covered categories (usu-ally on the basis of cost or cost-effectiveness considerations). A third level of decision concerns indications: for what conditions is the drug to be used? Finally, there may be 'drug use' decisions, including limits on the amount that might be prescribed for an episode.

Different types of reasons tend to be prominent at the four levels of decision. At the categorical and indication levels, for example, reasons range quite broadly over the goals of the plan (e.g. offering treatments but not 'medically unnecessary' enhance-ments), safety and efficacy, risk–benefit evaluations, and costs and cost-effectiveness. At the 'drug selection' and 'drug use' levels, decisions are more influenced by cost and cost-effectiveness than by other considerations.

These formulary design decisions all provide a context in which decision makers should be held accountable for the reasonable-ness of their decisions. They provide a perfect context in which a PBM company, in conjunction with the purchasers who contract for its services, can articulate a coherent framework of reasons and rationales that all fair-minded stakeholders can judge for their acceptability. These reasons and rationales, incorporated in the formulary design, then constitute a publicly accessible body of 'case law'. The 'case law' then helps the plan to remain consistent and coherent in its decision making and provides an educational device that can be used to help clinicians and patients in their deliberations about care.

Without an approach such as this, formulary design will be viewed as another 'bottom line' exercise, regardless of how much patient-oriented thought goes into deliberation about its features. Since pharmaceutical manufacturers more and more advertise directly to consumers, and since patients more and more have access to information on the Internet, PBM must be able to address the demand in a manner that reveals commitments, reasons and rationales that fair-minded participants in schemes, including clinicians, can see are relevant to meeting a population's health needs.

All stakeholders in our system, including large purchasers, such as employers, would benefit from insisting on accountability for reasonableness. If employers do not demonstrate a concern for the quality of the care they purchase, and if they are more and more seen only to be concerned about reducing costs, then the stability of the system will be undermined and the demand for intrusive – and perhaps cost-ineffective – regulation will increase.

Physician incentives

Accountability for reasonableness must be demanded and provided not only for direct limit setting, but also for indirect limit setting. More and more physicians have agreed to work under financial incentives aimed at limiting care and its cost (Gold *et al.* 1995). Most commonly, the health plan 'withholds' some percentage of the income of an otherwise fee-for-service provider, restoring the 'withhold' if organizational cost targets are achieved. With increasing frequency, physician groups, often those with the least familiarity with the cost-conscious culture of traditional, staff-model HMOs, accept the insurance risk of providing some range of patient services within a negotiated payment per patient per month. This capitation can also be coupled with bonuses and other incentives to reduce costs or achieve certain quality goals.

Do these novel incentives impose an undue risk on patients that physicians will violate the 'primacy principle', which calls on them to put patient welfare above their own financial interests? We do know, after all, that physicians respond to incentives (Hellinger

1996a; Orentlicher 1996). They modify their utilization of services in response to withholds and capitation schemes, and they do so not only in primary care settings, but in various specialty groups as well. If they do so respond, how can we be assured that these schemes do not impose unacceptable risks on patients? Accountability for reasonableness requires assurance to patients – evidence and arguments – that the incentive schemes negotiated between physicians and plans constitute a reasonable limit-setting device.

This test of reasonableness is illustrated by considering an important reason why simple disclosure of physician incentives, a measure called for in various codes of ethics for managed care and by proponents of 'market accountability', inadequately addresses the problem of 'conflict of interest' and the normative question about trust. If the only problem we face is identifying a hidden conflict of interest, then simple disclosure has some plausibility. But the real problem is more complex.

The real problem involves finding incentives that properly align and balance the several interests that are at stake in co-operative schemes to deliver health care. For example, because we are concerned in such schemes about population health and not simply the health of individual patients, we must also consider the interests of all parties in the covered population. Doctors cannot ignore the issue of population health, since they ration their own time and often must make implicit comparisons among their own patients. In addition, the private organizations, including for-profits, that organize and deliver care in our system acquire their own interests. These interests may also conflict with the interests of the covered populations as well as with the interests of the physicians that contract with them.

A reimbursement method such as capitation must achieve an appropriate, reasonable balance among these competing interests. This balance must seem reasonable to all fair-minded parties co-operating in these schemes in light of their common goal of meeting the health care needs of a covered population fairly under reasonable resource constraints. One implication is that fair-minded parties should recognize a collective interest in pursuing the cost-effective delivery of services. They should admit that reasonable resource constraints preclude providing every beneficial service regardless of cost.

If cost-effectiveness is relevant to pursuing population goals in health care, then incentives that push physicians to think about cost-effectiveness by giving them some direct interest in pursuing it may involve a *conflict of interest* with *individual* patients. At the same time, these incentives represent an *alignment of interests* between a *population* of patients and the physicians that treat them. Where multiple interests are at stake, the perception of conflict depends on perspective.

Of course, the economic incentives to physicians to undertreat could be too strong. This situation would come about if physicians and health plans form an alliance to share the benefits of reducing costs without careful consideration of the interests of the covered population. Physician interests would then conflict both with those of their individual patients and those of the population of patients as a whole.

A reasonable reimbursement method, then, must solve a complex problem in which interests may conflict in several directions. A reasonable solution should not, however, simply be the result of bargaining that reflects the relative power of the different interests – and the absence of patients from the table. It must be based on a consideration of how to achieve the common goal shared by fair-minded parties in the health care 'game'.

Existing guidelines for incentive schemes are based on theory, not evidence. Several authors (Berwick 1996; Pearson *et al.* 1998) have urged that incentive schemes should not put too much of a physician's income at risk and that risks should be spread over appropriately large groups of patients and physicians. But these recommendations – reasonable as they seem – should be backed by evidence that particular incentive arrangements do not put patients at undue risk. The main empirical study that focuses on this issue directly is a survey of the beliefs of plan managers about when they feel uncomfortable with the effects of incentives on clinicians (Daniels 1986). There is also no outcomes evidence to validate these beliefs.

It is simply not reasonable to put trust in the doctor–patient relationship at such risk without being able to show, through actual evidence, that incentive schemes are compatible with delivering appropriate care. Plans must provide institutional support for professional ethical values by providing not only disclosure, but actual evidence that their schemes are reasonable.

LEARNING ABOUT LIMITS IN THE LONG RUN

It is often remarked that Americans are particularly demanding, even individualistic, and that culturally they cannot accept the kinds of limits that might be imposed in less market-driven systems. People who make this remark use it to explain, in part, why Americans assign such a large role to the market in our system. The point can be turned around. Exposure to a market, rather than to a politically based system, can encourage irresponsible demand that ignores reasonable resource limits. In reality, however, resource limits are set, if only by employers and government purchasers. Consequently, there is all the more need for our society to embark on a learning process about health care limits.

There is no short-term solution to the problem of getting Americans (or others) to accept resource limits in health care. These limits will always seem arbitrary and unacceptable if the public thinks they are imposed by stakeholders with narrow economic interests. Suppose, however, that health plans demonstrate, through being held accountable for reasonableness, that they are making responsible decisions aimed at the shared goal of meeting needs fairly under resource constraints. Then there is the potential for an education in which the public internalizes conceptions of fair play that will moderate demand. Of course, people faced with life and death issues that affect their children or parents will try to do the most they can to help them. Whether they see restrictions as reasonable and fair, however, has a lot to do with their willingness to comply with them, even when their individual interests are threatened. There is no reason to think Americans are less amenable to fair play than the rest of the developed world.

The educative and deliberative role attributed to accountability for reasonableness is no less important elsewhere in the world. In many developing countries, as different as Chile, Colombia and Thailand, recent health care reforms have added significant private sector insurance schemes. These systems will inherit all the problems of legitimacy I have said are endemic in the United States.

Even in public systems or publicly administered systems, the problem of legitimacy arises. Accountability for reasonableness sets a standard for both the transparency of decision making and the grounds on which decisions are made. If adhered to, it would help transform what has often been a schizophrenic culture: though there is public accountability for the management of the health care system, and though in some countries general principles for the governance of these systems have been proclaimed, much decision making is done behind closed doors in the 'black box' of the budget at a local level. Accountability for reasonableness requires transparency about the grounds for these decisions. It also requires that the grounds should be generally accepted as relevant to meeting needs fairly under the budgetary constraints.

Accountability for reasonableness offers a way to resolve the controversy about implicit vs explicit rationing. Advocates of implicit rationing suggest that decisions are often quite complex and should not be reduced to some set of rigid rules given in advance. Doing so only ties the hands of experienced experts who can often make better decisions just by 'muddling through' and not raising the contentious problems that come from having to agree ahead of time on explict rules for rationing or limit setting. Advocates of explicit approaches argue it is important to provide a publicly acceptable, rational framework for these decisions, in part because we want to avoid the inconsistency that might result from leaving decisions to local 'experts' as they see fit. If the framework of rules is publicly agreed upon, then we also establish legitimacy for the decision makers.

Accountability for reasonableness suggests a middle path. In contrast to what explicitness seems to require, we may not be in a position to articulate a prior public consensus on principles or rules. In fact, we may need to develop such a consensus about acceptable, reason-governed practices in the process of making actual decisions. Over time, we can then articulate (through a form of 'case law') our commitments to the reasons that we agree are acceptable or relevant. In effect, we may have to 'muddle through' in some of our decision making. But, unlike the requirements of implicitness, we are held to a standard of public accountability that is more in the spirit of explicitness. Our reasoning while we 'muddle through' must be held up for scrutiny and public discussion, and we must be accountable for revising it in light of that discussion. We must seek decisions all can agree rest on reasonable considerations.

CONCLUSION

All health care systems must make morally controversial decisions that limit access to potentially beneficial medical services. Resistance to these decisions in the United States, as well as in publicly financed or administered systems, poses a challenge to the moral authority or legitimacy of decision makers. By holding health plans accountable for the reasonableness of their decisions it is possible to address this challenge. Accountability for reasonableness involves providing publicly accessible rationales for decisions and limiting rationales to those that all 'fair-minded' persons can agree are relevant to meeting patient needs fairly under resource constraints. This form of accountability provides a middle ground in the debate about 'explicit' vs 'implicit' forms of rationing.

ACKNOWLEDGEMENTS

James Sabin and I conducted the research on which this chapter is based with funding from the Greenwall Foundation, Retirement Research Foundation, National Science Foundation, Robert Wood Johnson Foundation, and the Harvard Pilgrim Health Care Foundation; I also acknowledge the assistance of a Robert Wood Johnson Investigator Award for Health Policy in preparing this chapter. We greatly appreciate the assistance of our research assistant, Roxanne Fay, for help in preparing earlier papers from which material for this was drawn.

10

TRAGIC CHOICES IN HEALTH CARE: LESSONS FROM THE CHILD B CASE

Chris Ham

In 1995 the case of Jaymee Bowen, more commonly known as Child B, captured the newspaper headlines. This case saw the coming together of a father who was determined to seek the treatment he believed was best for his daughter, doctors who disagreed about what treatment was appropriate, health service managers who were prepared to take a stand on the use of resources on services of questionable effectiveness, lawyers willing to test the decision of the health authority in the courts, and journalists who saw the case as exemplifying the dilemmas of health service decision making, ensuring that Jaymee's story caught the public imagination and highlighting the challenge of rationing (Ham and Pickard 1998). It also illustrated the conflict between a concern to respond to the needs of a patient with a life-threatening medical condition and a desire to use scarce health service resources for the benefit of the population as a whole. The way in which the case was handled by the health authority contains important lessons for those charged with making tragic choices in health care.

JAYMEE'S STORY

To understand the significance of the case it is important to recount some of the detail of what happened at the time. Jaymee Bowen was an articulate and lively child who was diagnosed as suffering from non-Hodgkin's lymphoma in 1990 at the age of 6. She was treated at Addenbrooke's Hospital in Cambridge but in 1993 was diagnosed as having a second cancer, acute myeloid leukaemia. Jaymee underwent chemotherapy and a bone marrow transplant for the treatment of her leukaemia at the Royal Marsden Hospital in London. Only nine months later, at the beginning of 1995, she relapsed, and the paediatricians responsible for her care advised that she had between six and eight weeks to live. Their view was that a child with Jaymee's medical history was unlikely to benefit from further intensive treatment and they recommended palliative care as the preferred option.

Jaymee's father, David Bowen, was not willing to accept this advice. His response to the opinions expressed by the doctors at Addenbrooke's and the Royal Marsden was to do his own research in the hope of finding a cure. As time was of the essence, he short-circuited most of the standard routines, making his own arrangements to seek medical advice, using faxes and phones, and working long hours on Jaymee's behalf to investigate alternative methods of treatment. David did this by reading books and medical journals, using his brother who lived in the United States, and contacting doctors at home and in hospital. The fact that he needed little sleep – no more than four hours a night – was particularly helpful in making contact with specialists in other time zones. His search eventually led to California where he found two doctors who were willing to recommend that Jaymee should receive a second bone marrow transplant.

David Bowen presented the results of his research to the paediatricians in the UK responsible for Jaymee's care. They were surprised that the specialists who had been contacted in California had recommended further intensive treatment in the light of Jaymee's medical history and the paucity of research into the outcomes of second transplants. Whereas their own view was that Jaymee's chances of going into remission following chemotherapy were around 10 per cent, with a similar probability that a second transplant would be successful, the advice from the US was much more optimistic. The paediatricians reiterated their opinion that palliative care was the best way of improving Jaymee's quality of life, emphasizing also that on balance the potential harm involved in chemotherapy and a second transplant outweighed the potential benefit. Their experience of treating similar cases had led them to be cautious in undertaking heroic interventions in the final stages of life and they were therefore not willing to acquiesce to David Bowen's request that they should proceed with a transplant.

At this point David arranged to see an adult leukaemia specialist at the Hammersmith Hospital on the advice of the experts from outside the UK with whom he had been in contact. The view of this specialist was much more positive. He put Jaymee's chances of going into remission following chemotherapy at 20 per cent, at which point a second transplant could be considered. Heartened by this opinion, David Bowen approached the Cambridge and Huntingdon Health Authority to ask if it would pay for treatment at the Hammersmith Hospital. The authority declined. Its director of public health argued that the paediatricians who had been responsible for Jaymee's care were in the best position to assess treatment options. In its view further intensive treatment was not appropriate in Jaymee's case and the authority was not prepared to use resources on experimental procedures with a limited chance of success. The health authority gave the same response when David Bowen presented the opinion of a leukaemia specialist working in the private sector that further treatment should be undertaken.

Reaching the end of the available options, David Bowen contacted his solicitors to seek leave for judicial review to challenge the authority's decision. This was granted and with legal aid in place preparations were made for the court proceedings. The High Court took the view that the health authority should reconsider its decision, arguing that the right to life was so precious that the authority should think again even though the chances of success were acknowledged to be low. This judgement was overturned on appeal. The judges in the Appeal Court, reaffirming the reluctance of the English courts to challenge health authority decisions on the funding of treatment, ruled that the authority had weighed the advice it had been given and that therefore there was no basis for the decision to be reviewed. By this stage the intense media interest in the case had made Child B headline news, in the process catapulting the health authority into the limelight. The decision not to fund a second transplant was analysed extensively in the press (Entwistle *et al.* 1996a), with the health authority being criticized in some newspapers for the stance it took. In response to media coverage an anonymous donor offered to provide funds for the treatment. David Bowen accepted this offer through his solicitors and treatment started in the private sector.

In the event, the specialist who took over Jaymee's care decided not to undertake a second transplant but instead used an experimental form of treatment known as donor lymphocyte infusion. He made this decision after consulting colleagues at an international conference and in the light of previous experience with other patients. This treatment enabled Jaymee to enjoy a few extra months of life. David Bowen believed that this vindicated the actions he had taken even though Jaymee became ill again and eventually died in May 1996. The fact that she had lived for over a year after the return of her leukaemia was diagnosed, much of this time with life of reasonable quality according to her father and the doctor in charge of her care, demonstrated the need to consider each case on its merits and to avoid treatment protocols which did not allow for the exceptions. In this respect, the consumerist challenge launched by David Bowen to the medical profession came to exemplify the increasing reluctance of patients and their families to accept that 'doctor always knows best' and the growing tendency for patients to seek further opinions until they receive the answer they want. For their part, the paediatricians who had looked after Jaymee continued to maintain that palliative care was the treatment of choice, a view supported by the health authority which paid for Jaymee's continuing care after her intensive treatment had come to an end.

THE ETHICS OF PRIORITY SETTING

Jaymee's story raises a series of ethical and practical issues of continuing relevance in the NHS. Most importantly, it demonstrates the tension between a concern to use resources for the benefit of the population as a whole and the urge to respond to the needs of individuals faced with the prospect of death. Although not motivated primarily by the costs of chemotherapy and a second transplant (estimated at £75,000), the Cambridge and Huntingdon Health Authority did take into account the likely benefit to be achieved from a significant financial outlay and the opportunity costs involved. In Jaymee's case, the combination of the high cost of treatment and the low chances of a successful outcome, against a background of clinical opinion which advised against further intensive treatment, were decisive considerations. As the body responsible for taking a community perspective on health care needs, the health authority felt that further intensive treatment for Jaymee was not only a low priority but also was not appropriate because it was not recommended by the doctors who knew her best.

The balance of costs and benefits looked quite different from David Bowen's perspective in that the alternative to going ahead with a transplant was the prospect that Jaymee would die within a

matter of weeks. Even though he recognized he was 'taking a calculated gamble', as the father of a dying child he felt this was a chance
worth taking in what were desperate circumstances. Although
David Bowen did not use this language, he was unconsciously
invoking the 'rule of rescue' (Hadorn 1991) in seeking help for
Jaymee. This suggests that when individuals are suffering life-
threatening conditions there is an obligation to intervene even
when this may run counter to the concerns of the community as a
whole. This rule applies regardless of the expenditure involved. In
a different context, the rescue of Tony Bullimore from his upturned
boat in the South Atlantic illustrates how utilitarian considerations
may have to be sacrificed if the alternative is certain death for an
individual at risk. By extension, medical intervention to save the
lives of patients who would otherwise die is appropriate, even
though the resources involved might bring more health benefit if
used in other ways.

The ethical dilemmas faced by health authorities have been
reviewed by Draper and Tunna (1996) who note the challenge of
meeting the needs of all individuals with the resources available.
Although health authorities have a particular responsibility to
ensure justice in the allocation of these resources, they are also
expected to respect each individual as a person in his or her own
right. In a case such as that of Child B, Draper and Tunna comment:

> In adjudicating a special claim on resources, by an identifiable
> individual, who is likely to die quite quickly if resources are not
> forthcoming, commissioners may feel compelled to assist, even
> if they would not consider the small possibility to benefit worth
> the cost under other circumstances, perhaps where death is not
> imminent.
>
> (Draper and Tunna 1996: 44)

In Jaymee Bowen's case the arguments were more complex
because the view of the child cancer specialists was that the potential harm involved in the act of rescue was likely to exceed the
potential benefit. They were also concerned that David Bowen
wished to protect Jaymee from full knowledge of her condition
because he believed that the chances of a successful outcome
would be enhanced by keeping her happy and feeling positive. The
view of the paediatricians was that Jaymee, an intelligent and
mature 10-year-old, should have been involved in weighing up
alternative courses of action and understanding the risks entailed.
Because David Bowen was unwilling to allow this, the doctors

concerned felt it was incumbent on them to assess Jaymee's best interests and to advise accordingly. Their experience of witnessing the adverse effects of intensive treatment on children like Jaymee urged caution in offering anything other than palliative care and lay behind their judgement that it was the appropriateness of treatment that mattered, not its cost.

This left the Cambridge and Huntingdon Health Authority to reach a decision in circumstances in which adult cancer specialists viewed the balance between harm and benefit differently from the paediatricians. In taking on this role, the authority was guided by a set of values it had adopted to inform its work as the commissioner of health services for the local community. These values enabled the managers involved to test the options in relation to the impact on equity, appropriateness, effectiveness, efficiency, responsiveness and accessibility. Like the child cancer specialists involved in the case, the authority felt that the evidence on appropriateness and effectiveness was of particular significance in the decision not to proceed with a second transplant. The existence of these values was seen by the authority to have been crucial in assisting it to arrive at a choice which was rigorous and defensible. Not least, they provided a template against which to assess alternatives and as such helped to promote greater consistency in priority-setting decisions.

THE PROCESS OF DECISION MAKING

The wider significance of the Child B case lies in the lessons it holds for those responsible for making tragic choices in health care. Among these lessons, the implications for health authorities and other bodies in the position of weighing the needs of individuals and the interests of the community are particularly important. As we have noted, the Cambridge and Huntingdon Health Authority was ultimately successful in defending the legal challenge to its decision and felt that the ruling in the Court of Appeal vindicated the approach it had taken.

This approach centred on the use of a set of values to inform decisions of this kind and a thorough process within the authority for assessing the evidence and considering alternatives. In this process, the director of public health took the lead and discussed the case with the authority's chief executive and chairman. The head of administration was also involved and these individuals reviewed the medical advice and evidence available before deciding not to acquiesce to David Bowen's wishes. When the case came to court, the authority was able to demonstrate that it had considered the evidence carefully and that the decision was not simply the result of one individual's judgement. It was also able to show that it had kept careful records of the case and the advice sought from clinicians. For these reasons, the way in which the case was handled was seen as exemplary by the Department of Health, notwithstanding the criticism directed at the authority by sections of the media.

Yet in making this point, it is important not to underestimate the scope for improving the process of decision making in cases of this kind. Given that there will often be controversy over tragic choices in health care, it is incumbent on those responsible for decision making to demonstrate that they have followed due processes and have been both rigorous and fair in arriving at their decisions. This is especially so in cases like that of Child B where an individual's life is at stake and when standard therapies have been exhausted. In this context, the research carried out by Daniels and Sabin (1997) into decisions on the funding and provision of new technologies in managed care organizations in the United States offers an interesting parallel to experience in the United Kingdom. Despite fundamental differences in the health care systems of these two countries, the ethical and practical dilemmas involved in decisions on the use of medical technologies are remarkably similar. As Daniels and Sabin argue, in circumstances in which patients and their relatives may fear that treatment is being denied on the basis of cost, decision makers have to be able to demonstrate that this is not the case if they are to invest the decision-making process with legitimacy.

Put another way, decision makers have to ensure 'accountability for reasonableness' (Daniels and Sabin 1998a) in decisions on health care coverage. Specifically, and in the context of managed care organizations, Daniels and Sabin propose four conditions that need to be met to ensure accountability for reasonableness. These are: .

1 *Publicity condition:* decisions regarding coverage for new technologies (and other limit-setting decisions) and their rationales must be publicly accessible.
2 *Relevance condition:* these rationales must rest on evidence, reasons and principles that all fair-minded parties (managers, clinicians, patients, and consumers in general) can agree are relevant to deciding how to meet the diverse needs of a covered population under necessary resource constraints.

3 *Appeals condition:* there is a mechanism for challenge and dispute resolution regarding limit-setting decisions, including the opportunity for revising decisions in light of further evidence or arguments.

4 *Enforcement condition:* there is either voluntary or public regulation of the process to ensure that the first three conditions are met.

(Daniels and Sabin 1998a: 57)

The approach taken by the Cambridge and Huntingdon Health Authority met some of these conditions but not others. For example, it could be argued that the application of a set of values to the Child B case met the relevance condition, but the way in which the authority's decision was communicated only partly fulfilled the publicity condition. On the latter point, more effort could have been made to explain the basis of the decision not to fund intensive treatment in advance of media attention and beyond the circle of those directly involved. Similarly, the appeals condition was not met in that there was no mechanism for challenge and dispute resolution other than a request to the health authority to reconsider its decision. The absence of such a mechanism meant that legal action was the only formal recourse available to the Bowen family.

The enforcement condition was met through judicial review of the health authority's decision but the restrictive scope of such reviews in the English legal system meant that only some aspects of the process proposed by Daniels and Sabin were scrutinized by the courts. In particular, the courts looked only at the health authority's decision-making process and did not require an explanation or justification of the decision or an assessment of the evidence on which it was based. As Parkin has commented, this approach '... risks failing to reassure those directly affected by the results of such policies as are developed that their individual cases are receiving properly worked out and consistently applied consideration' (Parkin 1995: 877).

Underpinning these arguments is the view that the process of decision making would be strengthened if reasons or rationales for decisions had to be made public. Taking this further, Daniels and Sabin contend that one of the effects of making public reasons for funding decisions would be to establish a body of 'case law'. As they state, this

involves a form of institutional reflective equilibrium. The considered judgements reflected in past decisions constitute relatively fixed points that can be revised only with careful deliberation and good reasons. Overall, there is a commitment to coherence in the giving of reasons – decisions must fit with each other in a plausible, reasonable and principle-mediated way . . .

A commitment to the transparency that case-law requires improves the quality of decision-making. An organization whose practice requires it to articulate explicit reasons for its decisions becomes focused in its decision-making.

(Daniels and Sabin 1997: 327–8)

The potential benefits include not only increased accountability for decision making but also greater consistency in the decision-making process. The advocates of such an approach maintain that openness would enhance public understanding of the necessity of priority-setting decisions and would foster a culture of education and learning between clinicians and patients (Daniels and Sabin 1997).

To make these points is to underscore the parallels between decision-making processes in health care and in the legal system. These parallels have been drawn out by Hadorn (1992) in the United States context in a way which reinforces the conclusions of this analysis. As Hadorn notes: 'The need to make relatively consistent case-by-case decisions amidst profound complexity is clearly one of the forces that has driven the health care system to adopt quasi-judicial features' (Hadorn 1992: 83). Like Daniels and Sabin, Hadorn argues that consistent procedures need to be adopted in health care and he contends that these procedures should be centred on the consideration of evidence concerning the outcomes of care, and the formulation of judgements based on this evidence. Continuing the analogy with the legal system, Hadorn suggests that judgements should be based on a standard of proof which might be more or less stringent depending on resource availability and the views of policy makers. The point emphasized here is that 'in the selection of a standard of proof . . . the fundamental balance between individual claims of need (that is, pursuit of individual good) and the greater public good is achieved' (Hadorn 1992: 83).

Applied to the Child B case, it could be argued that the Cambridge and Huntingdon Health Authority considered the evidence concerning outcomes, and decision makers in the authority used their judgement to arrive at a decision based on this evidence. In the process, the consideration given to the probability of intensive treatment being successful was an attempt to apply a standard of proof to the case, albeit implicitly. To this extent, the authority was conforming to the due process procedures advocated by Hadorn although, as we have seen, it is possible to identify aspects of these procedures that could be strengthened using the accountability for reasonableness conditions suggested by Daniels and Sabin.

CONCLUSION

While it is always hazardous to generalize from individual experiences, the case of Child B attracted such widespread attention and illustrated so many of the dilemmas of health service decision making that it would be an oversight not to seek to learn from the case and to draw out lessons for those who may be faced with similar dilemmas in future. Among the many issues to emerge, this paper has concentrated on the ethics of priority setting and the process of decision making. It has demonstrated that the Cambridge and Huntingdon Health Authority gained credit for the way in which it handled the case, its experience serving as an example from which others can learn. At the same time, aspects of the decision-making process could have been strengthened, most obviously through the giving of reasons for the decision and the establishment of an appeals mechanism. The reason for emphasizing the need to improve the process of decision making is that cases of this kind are always likely to generate debate and disagreement. What therefore matters is to structure the debate to enable different points of view to be articulated, to promote transparency and consistency in decision making, and to build trust, confidence and legitimacy in the process. In the longer term, these characteristics of due process in decision making should enhance public understanding of choices in health care and promote more informed discussion of the issues.

ACKNOWLEDGEMENTS

Thanks are due to the King's Fund which supported the research on which this chapter is based, all of those who were interviewed during the research, and Susan Pickard who worked with me in carrying out the research and co-authored the book on which this chapter is based.

11

FAIRNESS AS A PROBLEM OF LOVE AND THE HEART: A CLINICIAN'S PERSPECTIVE ON PRIORITY SETTING

James E. Sabin

From the clinician's perspective cost-effectiveness analyses and priority-setting exercises are highly abstract compared with the experience of taking care of patients. We encounter the ill person directly, convey the priorities, and deal with the impact on patient and family. For those of us who take direct care of patients, priorities and rationing – at their deepest level – create what is ultimately a problem of love and the heart.

To be truly excellent clinicians we must love our patients, and that makes us want to do as much as possible for each person's health. To be truly responsible citizens, however, we must want to do as much as possible for the population's health within the available resources. This commitment to fairness requires us to embrace priorities and rationing. In the United States we call love for patients fidelity, and seeking fairness for the population stewardship. Since priority setting and rationing inevitably deprive identifiable people of potential benefits, the question for practising clinicians is whether they can embrace fidelity and stewardship at the same time in their dealings with patients.

I believe the answer is yes, and disagree with Kassirer's recent argument that doctors should not adopt a population-based ethic (Kassirer 1998). Embracing both fidelity and stewardship, however, poses at least as much challenge to the heart as to the mind.

Correspondingly, the four-step analysis that follows emphasizes passion as well as logic.

Box 11.1 Combining passion and logic

- Priority setting and rationing will not work without the support of clinicians.
- Ethical clinicians can (and should) accept fair priority and rationing policies.
- Implicit rationing is not a viable strategy for the twenty-first century.
- Societies must deliberate about how to make priorities and rationing work best.

CLINICAL SUPPORT FOR RATIONING

Political leadership is a key factor in helping the public to understand the need for priorities and rationing. In the United States Dr John Kitzhaber, now the governor of Oregon, was crucial in helping Oregon carry out its justifiably famous priority-setting process. But clinicians are at least as important as political leaders in shaping public attitudes. Every clinical appointment, whether with a general practitioner, a specialist or a district nurse, is an opportunity for patients to learn about priorities and rationing and for clinicians to learn what these policies mean in their patients' lives.

When we clinicians support policies about priorities and rationing we can be educators and salespeople. But when we oppose the policies we can undermine them and foment resistance. We may not always be wise in our judgements, but no national approach to priorities and rationing will work without our strong support.

FAIR PRIORITY AND RATIONING POLICIES

On the clinical front line we ask ourselves: are these priorities ethical for the patient who is in front of me now? How can I discuss the policy openly and honestly? To be able to practise in a health system that sets priorities and rations we need a professional ethic that can give us guidance for these questions.

The United States provides a useful test case here. It probably has the world's strongest culture based on individual rights. It certainly has the least inclusive health care system among developed nations. However, an experience at the health maintenance organization I have practised with for 23 years taught me that even in a culture as individualistic as that in the United States clinicians and patients can understand and accept priorities and rationing if the rationale is clear and readily understandable.

Six years ago my colleagues in mental health – with the advice of the population we serve – concluded that we needed to offer more outpatient care to our sickest patients. Although we were not given any new money to do this, we were allowed to reorder our service's priorities. We concluded that we could increase services to our sickest patients only by requiring a new payment from the less sick after their eighth outpatient appointment (Abrams 1993).

After we made this change my colleagues and I had innumerable conversations with our patients about the new policy. With patients who were eligible for more services we said something like, 'The bad news, as we know, is that you have the misfortune of suffering from a severe illness (schizophrenia or a similar severe ailment). The good news is that we now have more outpatient treatment resources available to us!' With our healthier patients, who now had to make a payment after eight outpatient sessions, we had the opposite conversation: 'The good news is that even though you have some significant problems you do not have a severe illness like schizophrenia or manic depression. The bad news is that after eight sessions there is now a new fee.' No one thought that the policy was unfair.

We did not explain the priority system by presenting cost-effectiveness analyses or complex ethical arguments. We used simple, commonsense terms that made fundamental human sense. The policy had the same kind of obvious reasonableness as when we interrupt an appointment with one patient to attend to an emergency with another.

To support priorities and rationing, clinicians must be able to see the policy rationale with the same emotional clarity and immediacy with which we see our individual patients' needs. To explain the policy we must be able to put it in simple terms that do not presuppose a university degree in economics or philosophy.

We clinicians can love our patients and the population they are part of only when we can comprehend the needs of both in emotional as well as clinical and epidemiological terms. Being able to do this depends partly on whether our clinical education and professional ethics include public health as well as individual care values (Sabin 1994). But it depends at least as much on a political process that addresses priorities and rationing in the same caretaking spirit that the best clinicians apply in the care of their patients. This requires a form of political leadership that has been comparatively rare to date.

IMPLICIT RATIONING IS NOT VIABLE

Although I strongly support openness about priorities and rationing, there are two strong arguments for implementing them implicitly – that is, not discussing them in the clinician–patient relationship (Mechanic 1995).

First, withholding benefits is socially divisive. Being explicit about priorities and rationing requires acknowledging that there are good things that a health care system could do for identifiable people that it will not do (Calabresi and Bobbitt 1978). In the United Kingdom explicitness leads to shroud waving. In the United States it leads to lawsuits. Neither is pleasant for policy makers.

Second, patients (and clinicians) prefer to see clinicians as giving, not withholding. We clinicians chose our careers to care for patients, not to implement priorities. And sick patients need to see their clinicians as devoted caretakers, not as coldly utilitarian cost-effectiveness analysts.

Since the kinds of expectations patients in the United States have about disclosure and active participation in treatment planning almost certainly predict the worldwide trend for the next century, the United States can provide useful lessons about implicit rationing. Fifty years ago the phrase 'doctor's orders' was used with great seriousness. What the doctor said, the patient did. Now we use the term only in quotation marks, as a quaint and humorous relic. Patients in the United States expect to be told the medical facts about their conditions and the policy facts about what the health care system will and will not do for them.

Personal computers and the Internet drive the nails into the coffin of implicit rationing. The Internet gives patients access to worldwide information about health care policies and choices. This means that within a short time implicit rationing will be impossible. Explicitness is the inevitable direction for priorities and rationing. Clinicians and political leaders will be wise to shape the process rather than waiting to have it forced on them. I believe that this is the best climate for practice. But even if it is not it is nevertheless the direction all societies will be moving in.

HOW TO MAKE RATIONING WORK

Setting health care priorities and rationing is an unavoidably messy, conflict-ridden, ultimately tragic social process (Calabresi and Bobbitt 1978). Different societies will conduct the process in accord with their own political culture. But whatever approach a society chooses, it is not likely to succeed without some form of deliberation among the concerned stakeholders (Daniels and Sabin 1998a).

We in the United States have conducted a social experiment in which we tried to shape health care without explicit priorities or deliberative process. Motivated by the reluctance of the medical profession to accept the need for priorities and rationing, and the conviction held by influential physicians that ethical clinicians must advocate any intervention of possible benefit to their patients (Levinsky 1984), the United States has experimented with what is best described as an adversarial system of priority setting. We have asked our insurance companies – the United States version of district health authorities – to set priorities for us.

Here is how the adversarial form of managed care works. Physicians recommend services for their patients. Insurers decide whether the service will be covered. Physicians act as pure advocates. Insurers make decisions in the light of the available funds. Physicians hold to fidelity. Insurers take care of stewardship.

The experience of the United States shows that this adversarial approach results in a high degree of public distrust of the system itself (Blendon *et al.* 1998). How could it be otherwise? Since patients largely trust their clinicians then of course they distrust a system in which their clinicians petition the insurer for coverage and get turned down. Whether or not the insurance decisions and policies can be justified by ethical reasoning and cost-effectiveness analyses, splitting fidelity from stewardship and placing them in opposing camps invites patients to see their clinicians as impotent and the system as unfair. A system that splits fidelity from stewardship simply doesn't work.

The American system commits itself to providing medically necessary treatment. We have skirted, however, the fundamental question of how to define medical necessity. Is any intervention that physicians believe will benefit their patients medically necessary?

Many doctors define the term this way. Does medically necessary mean worthwhile in the light of the available resources and needs of the population? Many insurers define the term more like this. Except in the state of Oregon, however, the United States has had no open debate on what standards we will use for necessity in medical practice. In the absence of debate, the public, sensing the wide disparity among definitions and realizing that unacknowledged rationing decisions are being made, has responded with anger, cynicism and distrust.

To create the necessary dialogue about priorities and rationing, societies must learn how to do what a popular book on corporate management calls 'replacing the tyranny of the OR with the genius of the AND' (Collins and Porras 1997). American clinicians call the managers who concern themselves with budgets and priorities bean counters. A British physician told me that management is the syphilis of the NHS. I am sure that clinicians from other countries can add choice terms in other languages. And I am equally sure that managers have just as many disparaging terms for clinicians.

Until clinicians, managers and other stakeholders find a common language for deliberating together about priorities and rationing, we cannot expect the public to understand and accept limit-setting policies (Sabin 1992).

CONCLUSION

I believe that our path towards societal resolution of the conflicts between individual and community needs and desires demands more of the heart than the brain. Clinicians are inextricably in the midst of these conflicts. Our distress with priorities and rationing must be understood as crucial data on a social process, not as resistance to be overcome. Patients and society need clinicians to love both the individual and the collective and need to join with them in deliberating about solutions to this painful but ultimately unavoidable conflict of the heart. The key requirements are an expanded health care ethic (Berwick *et al.* 1997) and courageous political leadership.

ACKNOWLEDGEMENTS

This chapter was originally published in the *British Medical Journal* of 10 October 1998, 317, 1002–4, reproduced with kind permission.

12

THE ETHICS OF DECENTRALIZING HEALTH CARE PRIORITY SETTING IN CANADA

John R. Williams and Michael Yeo

In this chapter[1] we describe and analyse, from the standpoint of ethics, a consistent national strategy for delegating the responsibility for health care priority setting to regional authorities. We begin with a brief overview of the recent decentralization of health care in Canada. We then deal with the ethical issues raised by decentralization of priority setting for governments, regional boards, regional staff, health care providers and the public. We conclude with some suggestions for addressing these issues.

The authors, individually and collectively, conducted ethics workshops for regional health authorities in three Canadian jurisdictions: Prince Edward Island (Williams *et al.* 1996; Yeo *et al.* 1998), Alberta, and the Northwest Territories, between 1995 and 1997. Preparations for these workshops involved extensive review of the literature on health care reform, governance and priority setting. The workshops themselves provided qualitative data on the difficulties encountered by regional authorities in setting priorities and on the solutions they have devised for dealing with these problems. The authors analysed this experience in the light of the literature, including materials published subsequently.

BACKGROUND

Since the formation of Canada in 1867, health care has been a provincial responsibility. However, for almost 50 years the federal government has provided funding for hospital and physician services through the national health insurance plan, Medicare, under conditions set forth most recently in the Canada Health Act of 1984. During the 1990s, in order to deal with large budgetary deficits, the federal government unilaterally reduced its fiscal transfers to the ten provincial and two territorial governments for health care. In response, the provinces and territories sought new ways to economize on health care spending. One such strategy was decentralization or, as it is more commonly termed, 'regionalization'.

Between 1992 and 1996 health care was regionalized in every province of Canada except Ontario, and in the Northwest Territories (Lomas *et al.* 1997a). The stated reasons for adopting this strategy were similar in all jurisdictions:

- it brings services 'closer to home' in that it allows communities to identify their own priorities for health services and to participate more fully in the delivery of these services;
- it increases accountability in health care by connecting more closely the decision makers (i.e. the regional boards) and those affected by the decisions; and
- it allows senior governments (federal and provincial) to reduce overall expenditure on health care without incurring the displeasure of the electorate since the actual programme cuts are made at the regional level.

The mandate of regional authorities varies from province to province. Prince Edward Island boards have the broadest mandate, which includes not only health services but social services such as social assistance and corrections. Quebec boards deal with health and community support services and social assistance; Newfoundland and New Brunswick boards deal only with hospitals and nursing homes. The other jurisdictions deal with a broad range of health but not social services.

The powers that have been devolved to regional authorities include, but are not limited to, priority setting. The authorities are also responsible for local planning, allocating funds and managing services (Lomas *et al.* 1997a: 373). In this chapter we will focus on their role in setting priorities.

Although regionalization has been extolled as a means of

decentralizing power and authority from the province to more local groups, it has also had the opposite effect of removing power and authority from many hospital and community health services boards and centralizing it at the regional level. This has been done in the name of efficiency but it seems to go against the principle of community empowerment. Furthermore, wherever regionalization has occurred, the senior government has been very reluctant to give up its power to determine overall funding and to override the decisions of regional boards.

The first members of regional boards across the country were all appointed by government. Many jurisdictions announced their intention to move eventually to elected boards, but so far this has happened only in Saskatchewan. Both selection processes raise important ethical issues, which we discuss below.

ETHICAL ISSUES

In dealing with the ethical issues raised by the regionalization of priority setting, we first of all have to clarify what we mean by an ethical issue.

> An issue involves conflict and controversy. *Ethical* issues bear upon the rights and wrongs of human decision making and behaviour. They involve conflicting beliefs about how human beings should live, about the values individuals and groups should uphold, and about the values that may be sacrificed when all values in a situation cannot be honoured and maintained. Issues in *bioethics* centre upon right and wrong decisions, policies and acts in medicine and healthcare and in the uses of biomedical science and technology.
>
> (Roy *et al.* 1994: 30)

There are two general types of ethical issues: substantive and procedural. With the former the outcome sought is a good answer, decision or policy. This requires asking questions such as which ends or goals should be pursued and which should be avoided, and which means should be used to attain these goals and which should be avoided. Different procedures or processes can be used for choosing goals and means, some better and others worse. To ensure accountability as required in a democratic society, the process of public policy making, whether by governments or regional boards, should be transparent and open to scrutiny and should incorporate some degree of meaningful public participation. It should both be and be seen to be fair.

Health care priority setting involves *ethical* issues because it requires decisions about who should benefit when not all can, and the benefits at stake are health and well-being and sometimes even life itself. These are substantive issues, involving decisions about both the goals of health care and the means of attaining these goals. For example, should the first priority be to provide care for those who are injured or diseased or should it be to promote healthy and safe living to prevent injury and disease? What should be the balance between these two? For each of these goals there are many different means that can be used to attain it. On what basis should the choice among these means be made – the utilitarian principle of the greatest good for the greatest number? Priority to the most disadvantaged members of society? Allowing people to purchase better care for themselves?

In a pluralist society, it may be impossible to achieve meaningful consensus on many substantive issues. However, even if there is no 'right' answer, this does not mean that all answers are equally valid. Particularly in cases where consensus does not exist, decision makers should strive for 'morally defensible' decisions, that is, decisions for which all relevant considerations have been duly entertained and the justificatory reasons have been clearly laid out. If others do not accept the answer, they should at least understand and appreciate the reasons that led to it and be able to challenge it on grounds of principle. The process by which the decision is reached should therefore be transparent and open to scrutiny. Along these lines, health care priority setting raises numerous procedural issues, such as how decision makers are chosen or designated, what sort of consultation is undertaken and how decisions are communicated.

We will now describe the issues, both substantive and procedural, that regionalization of priority setting raises for the various decision makers: governments, regional boards, regional staff, health care providers and the public. The one group that is missing from this list, arguably the most important, is patients and their families. They are certainly affected by regionalization, but since they have little if any control over the process, we will not discuss them in this chapter.

Governments

As those ultimately responsible for the health care system and as the initiators of regionalization, provincial politicians and civil servants have taken upon themselves an enormous responsibility in promoting this type of change to the system. First of all, regionalization is basically an experiment, undertaken with no strong evidence that it will improve health care planning and delivery. Moreover, except in Prince Edward Island (PEI Health and Community Services System 1997a and 1997b), there has been no systematic attempt to evaluate the changes brought about by regionalization. Governments will always be able to point to some indicators to show that regionalization is successful, but many people will feel that they are worse off than before.

This difference between government and user perspectives requires government, as the more powerful of the two parties, to be transparent about how much power it intends to give up to the regional boards and whether it expects the boards to be accountable primarily to it or to the people of the region. If government is not willing to give the regional boards significant authority to determine priorities and allocate funds, then it should state this clearly, even if the result is that not many people are willing to serve on boards with such limited powers.

One related procedural issue for governments is whether to have board members appointed or elected. The goal is the same in either case – to get a high-quality, dedicated and representative board. There are advantages and disadvantages to each process that can be used to achieve this goal. Appointed boards may be less subject to pressure from interest groups, whether users of services, health care providers or local communities. Conversely, they may be less representative of the people in the region and less accountable to them. Members of elected boards will be likely to have defined constituencies, either geographical or sectoral (physicians, nurses, consumers, labour, etc.) for whom they can serve as advocates, but they may find it difficult to set priorities in the interests of the whole region for fear that they will not be re-elected by their constituents. When deciding this matter, government should seek to minimize the disadvantages of the process it chooses, for example by publicizing the criteria used to select members for appointment or by not making the job of elected board members so difficult that they will never be re-elected.

Regional boards

Priority setting raises important ethical issues, both substantive and procedural, for regional boards. The substantive issues include what health and health care goals to pursue and what means to choose for achieving these goals. The highest priority goal could be a reduction in sexually transmitted diseases, improved home care for elderly persons or decreased waiting times for cardiac surgery, among many others. The choice among these goals will involve consideration of ethical values such as fairness, compassion and relief of suffering. There will probably be a variety of means available to attain any one of these goals. For example, the reduction in sexually transmitted diseases could be achieved by improved sexuality education, by widespread distribution of condoms or by publicizing the identity of infected individuals. Here, too, choices are value-laden, and may require trade-offs between competing values such as parental responsibility for children and respect for privacy.

Regional boards must also deal with procedural issues in priority setting and resource allocation. Since these matters affect the people of the region, the people should have some real input to the board's decision-making process. The board should take this input seriously, even if it cannot agree to all the demands of the various stakeholders. And it should report back to the people the reasons for its decisions.

How should regional boards deal with these ethical issues? Ethics is just as much a field of expertise as economics and politics, and it is not to be expected that board members will come equipped with the necessary ethical competence. Some assistance will be needed; this can be obtained by establishing an ethics advisory committee, by hiring a staff person or consultant with training and experience in ethics, or by participating in a network to share ethics resources. Alberta has such a network.[2]

Regional staff

In most large organizations it is the staff who carry out the directions of the board. According to one popular model of organizational governance (Carver 1990) that has been adopted by several Canadian regional boards, the board's job is to determine the goals or ends to be pursued and the staff are free to choose the means for attaining these ends, subject to any specific limitations imposed by the board. In this model the staff need to be able to recognize and avoid means that are unethical. They also have to advise the board about the ethical pros and cons of different goals and about process issues. Clearly there is a need for ethical competence at the staff level.

As staff are transferred from local institutions to the regional authority, they may experience ethical conflicts between their loyalty to their former workplace and patients and their responsibility to the new, larger constituency. They may feel that their old institution and its patients or residents and staff are being treated unfairly when priorities are established for the new structure, and that it is their duty to rectify this unfairness even if it means going against the board's decisions. In such situations staff should have the opportunity to voice their concerns and to hear the rationale for board decisions if the board does not support their position.

Even if they experience no such conflicts, regional staff must still deal with other ethical issues in priority setting and rationing scarce resources. The board may set general policies for allocating resources, but the staff are often the ones who are faced with urgent demands for funds for very worthwhile programmes that cannot all be supported. For example, there may be tremendous pressure from family members, perhaps supported by the media, to pay for experimental treatment in another country for a dying child, even though the chances of success are low and the money required could provide proven benefits for a great many other children (for example, through a vaccination or school lunch programme). Refusing such requests can lead to charges of heartlessness and even cruelty, but giving in to them establishes precedents that can play havoc with carefully constructed priorities. Regional staff must learn how to deal with these difficult issues and need to be fully supported by their board.

Health care providers

Some of the strongest criticism of regionalization has come from the front-line providers of health care: doctors, nurses, chaplains, social workers and others. They have two main concerns: the effect of changes in the delivery of health care on their patients or clients, and on their own conditions of employment. The fact that regionalization has come into vogue at a time of cuts to health care budgets and that one of the main reasons for the changes is to achieve greater efficiencies has led many providers to conclude that the health and well-being of individual patients is not a high priority for government planners. This suspicion is reinforced by the widespread emphasis on health promotion, which many providers feel entails sacrificing those who are currently injured or sick in favour of a future, healthier population.

Providers also feel that they are disproportionately affected by regionalization and that they have very little input to the changes. Indeed, most provincial and territorial governments have either excluded or greatly restricted provider eligibility for membership of regional boards. As professionals used to exercising a great deal of control over their practices, some provider groups resent health priorities being determined by people who know far less than they do about the day-to-day realities of health care. They also fear a patchwork of regional employment policies across a province or territory in which their traditional bargaining agents, the provincial or territorial associations, have no authority. Some of these drawbacks of regionalization have so far been forestalled, as the senior governments have retained control over provider remuneration and in some places have developed standard staff agreements for all regions. However, since salaries account for a large proportion of regional budgets, providers fear that the next step in regionalization may be to give the regions authority over the remuneration and working conditions of providers. Where there is a 'buyer's market' for health professionals, this could lead to a deterioration of salaries and benefits and a consequent lowering of provider morale.

The public

If regionalization works according to plan, members of the public will have more control over their health, in that they will have a greater say in which programmes will be provided and where. If boards are elected, members of the public will have regular opportunities to indicate their agreement or disagreement with the board's priorities. However, with this greater control comes greater responsibility. People may have to decide which health services they will receive and which ones they will do without. If they want extra services, they will probably have to pay extra for them. The notion of 'free health care' or 'the government will pay for it' will become increasingly untenable.

Regionalization could also give members of the public an opportunity to form interest groups to pressure the board for special consideration. On the basis of 'the squeaky wheel gets the grease' principle, each community, disease or disability-specific group and provider organization can try to persuade the board and staff to favour its causes over others. Some might applaud this approach as evidence of a healthy democracy, but others would say that fairness can be a casualty of such interest group politics.

Does the public know what is good for it? This is a perennial question for health care planners and poses a dilemma for governments and regional boards. On the one hand, the principle of democracy would have the public decide for itself what it should have. On the other hand, the 'experts' feel that what the public wants is often different from what it really needs. In Prince Edward Island, regional officials discovered that the public continues to give highest priority to sickness care despite efforts to convince them that funds should be shifted to health promotion and disease prevention (Lomas and Rachlis 1996: 20). If regionalization gives the public a greater influence on setting priorities for health services, members of the public clearly have a responsibility to think carefully about the different options and their advantages and disadvantages. In the end, however, their values will determine what they think is most important, and if the regional boards believe in democracy, they will accept and implement the public's wishes. And to the extent that the public participates in decision making and influences policy decisions, the public should be adequately informed about the issues, including the trade-offs to be made (Yeo 1996). This means that regionalization should include some considerable budget for meaningful consultation and participation.

CONCLUSION

We have described some of the ethical issues raised by regionalization of health care priority setting. It is a formidable list, and it makes one wonder whether, if these had been thought about in advance, regionalization would ever have been initiated. Nevertheless, regionalizaton is well underway, and it would be very difficult at this stage to reverse the process. The ethical issues need to be faced and dealt with, in as explicit and systematic a manner as possible. But will this actually happen? The programme for evaluating regionalization in Prince Edward Island mentioned above is being implemented (PEI Health and Community Services System 1997a, 1997b). Unfortunately, the very elaborate questionnaires designed for this purpose ignore almost totally the ethical issues discussed here. Evidently the experts in charge of this programme are either oblivious to these issues or else consider them unimportant. Evaluations of regionalization in Alberta (Casebeer and Hannah 1998), Saskatchewan (Kouri *et al.* 1997; Borody and Gieni 1998) and across Canada (Lomas 1997a) suffer from the same defect.

All this is to say that those who feel that these issues are important will have to work hard to ensure that they receive the consideration they deserve. Here are some suggestions for how this might be done.

- Government officials, health care planners and regional boards and staff should be encouraged to identify and address the ethical issues of priority setting both before and during the implementation of regionalization.
- Regional boards should be encouraged to clarify the values and principles that guide their priority-setting work, as regards both the goals of health and health care and the means for attaining these goals.
- Decision making at all levels should be transparent and open to scrutiny; the reasons for decisions and the process for reaching them should be public so that decision makers can be held accountable.
- Public education programmes should be developed to prepare the public to participate in priority setting and to demand accountability from governments and regional boards for their choice of priorities.

NOTES

1 The opinions expressed in this chapter are those of the authors. They do not necessarily represent Canadian Medical Association policy.
2 The Alberta Provincial Health Ethics Network's website is:
http: //www.phen.ab.ca/home2.html

PART V

TECHNIQUES FOR DETERMINING PRIORITIES

13

PRIORITY SETTING AND HEALTH TECHNOLOGY ASSESSMENT: BEYOND EVIDENCE-BASED MEDICINE AND COST-EFFECTIVENESS ANALYSIS

Douglas K. Martin and Peter A. Singer

Imagine that you are the medical director of an organization responsible for coordinating cancer care in your province (or state). The government has decided to invest $11 million in new and emerging cancer drugs for the next year. You estimate that funding all possible new and emerging cancer drugs for your population in the next year would cost $50 million. How should you decide which drugs to fund for which patients?

Priority setting for new health technologies is a common problem in every developed country in the world. It is faced not only in primarily publicly funded systems, such as Canada or the UK, but also in primarily privately funded systems such as the USA. The medical director of a large HMO confronts precisely the same challenge as the medical director of the publicly funded cancer care agency described in the scenario.

Priority setting can be defined as the distribution of resources among competing programmes or people (McKneally *et al.* 1997). It occurs simultaneously at the macro (government), meso (hospital or institution), and micro (bedside) levels.

At the macro (health system) level, Deber *et al.* (1997) summarized five potential frameworks for priority setting including: the Canada Health Act approach; the Oregon Model; the Netherlands Four-Sieve Model; The Four-Screen Model; and the Canadian Medical Association Core and Comprehensiveness Project. Each of these frameworks addresses health care system priority setting but they are not specifically targeted at health technology assessment.

At the micro (bedside) level, an important unresolved question is what role physicians should play in priority setting. Two conflicting views have emerged:

1 'physicians are required to do everything that they believe may benefit each patient without regard to costs or other societal considerations' (Levinsky 1984: 1575); and
2 'the physician's obligations to the patient can no longer be a single-minded, unequivocal commitment but rather must reflect a balancing. Patients' interests must be weighed against the legitimate competing claims of other patients, of payers, of society as a whole, and sometimes even of the physician himself' (Morreim 1995: 2).

A detailed examination of priority setting at the macro or micro levels is beyond the scope of this chapter.

The focus of this chapter is on health technology assessment, which tends to occur in meso-level institutions in the health care system. Health technology assessment can be defined as 'the evaluation or testing of a medical technology for safety and efficacy. In a broader sense, it ... examines the short- and long-term consequences of individual medical technologies' (Office of Technology Assessment 1982: 3). The importance of priority setting in health technology assessment is well recognized. As Battista has written, 'We [should] situate technology assessment within a framework of responsible stewardship of resources' (Battista 1996). Moreover, some of the key case studies in health technology assessment of the last decade – for example, high vs low osmolar contrast media for radiological procedures, and streptokinase vs tissue plasminogen activator (TPA) for acute myocardial infarction – have driven home the point that priority setting is a key aspect of health technology assessment.

The purpose of this chapter is to review the current state of knowledge and propose a new research approach to priority setting and health technology assessment. In the second section we examine existing discipline-specific theoretical perspectives and their two main limitations – lack of empirical grounding and lack of inter-connections between perspectives. These two limitations become the focus of the next two sections. We describe relevant empirical studies, evaluate their limitations, and propose a research approach involving case study and grounded theory methods. We then examine unresolved priority-setting problems resulting from the lack of connections among and within discipline-specific theoretical perspectives, and propose a research approach using interdisciplinary methods. Finally, we consolidate the suggested approach to future research developed in the previous two sections, and illustrate how this approach may lead to a third phase of priority setting, reconciling the 'simple solutions' and 'muddling through' of the first and second stages of priority setting (Holm 1998; Klein 1998).

DISCIPLINE-SPECIFIC PERSPECTIVES ON PRIORITY SETTING

Philosophy, law, political science, medicine and economics each offer their own perspective on how priority-setting decisions should be made. This section will briefly review these perspectives before highlighting the problems with the discipline-specific approach.

Philosophy

Theories of distributive justice pertain to priority setting. Utilitarian theories emphasize the 'greatest good for the greatest number'. Egalitarian theories emphasize need and equality of opportunity. Libertarian theories emphasize the process by which resource allocation decisions are made. There is no theory of justice to resolve conflicting claims when the various theories lead to different conclusions.

Law

Three distinct legal issues arise concerning priority setting for health technologies: the right to health care, prohibitions against discrimination, and the obligations of the physician. First, countries with universal health coverage (e.g. the United Kingdom) have legislation mandating reasonable access to medically necessary services. Second, although it is often difficult to determine on what grounds resources should be allocated, international conventions such as the Universal Declaration of Human Rights and national constitutions prohibit discrimination on grounds including race, religion, age and sex. Third, and increasingly controversial, is the common law tradition that physicians' primary duty is to their patients, and that financial considerations cannot play a decisive role in clinical decisions.

Political science

A key element in priority setting is the 'fairness' of the decision-making process itself. Political science in particular has contributed useful conceptual frameworks for analysing allocation processes and the participation of stakeholders, including representatives of the public. There is also empirical evidence that lay decision makers may feel unqualified or unwilling to participate in health care priority-setting exercises (Klein 1993a; Lomas 1997b).

Medicine

Health care providers and health scientists use evidence-based medicine (EBM) to contribute to the understanding of effectiveness. EBM can be defined as 'the conscientious and judicious use of current best evidence from clinical care research in the management of individual patients' (Haynes *et al.* 1996). EBM helps to quantify, or categorize, benefits, harms and level of evidence so that providers and patients may choose an appropriately individualized treatment plan. It does not, however, balance effectiveness with other competing values such as cost.

Economics

Health economists have been predominantly concerned with the efficiency and equity of distributions of resources most often using the problematic concept of 'need' as the discriminating variable. Cost-effectiveness analysis (CEA) has been widely promoted as a tool for pursuing equitable and efficient investments in health care technologies (Tengs *et al.* 1995). However, the use of CEA remains controversial for a variety of philosophical and practical reasons, including its fundamental reliance on utilitarian reasoning and inability to incorporate other distributive justice principles. The Panel on Cost-Effectiveness in Health and Medicine recognized that '. . . CEA [should] be used as an aid to decision makers who must weigh the information it provides in the context of . . . other values' (Russel *et al.* 1996: 1177). Despite this caveat, it is fair to say that the last two perspectives – evidence-based medicine and cost-effectiveness analysis – have had the greatest influence on health technology assessment. To somewhat oversimplify the matter, the prevailing model of resource allocation in health technology assessment can be represented as: Δ Costs/Δ Benefits.

PROBLEMS WITH THE DISCIPLINE-SPECIFIC PERSPECTIVES APPROACH

How does this spectrum of discipline-specific perspectives, including the prevailing models of EBM and CEA, assist the medical director of the provincial cancer agency faced with the mandate to allocate $11 million of funding on a possible menu of $50 million of new and emerging cancer drugs? There are two main limitations in making the leap from discipline-specific perspectives to the challenge faced by the cancer agency medical director. First, the discipline-specific perspectives are not grounded in actual experiences of priority setting such as that faced by the cancer agency medical director. Second, there are few interconnections among the various discipline-specific perspectives (and even within each perspective – such as between different theories of justice). The next two sections will address each of these limitations in turn.

Grounding in actual experience

Currently, there is relatively little empirical research into the way actual decision-making bodies define, deliberate upon, and resolve the many issues involved in priority setting. Normative frameworks for 'rationing' decisions have been prescribed with surprisingly little appreciation of the values, interests, or reasoning styles of the decision makers who are supposed to apply them.

Surveys of health care professionals show that rationing is occurring, for example, in dialysis (Mendelssohn *et al.* 1995), critical care (SCCMEC 1994), cardiac care (Fleming *et al.* 1991), transplantation (Mullen *et al.* 1996), and possibly implicitly for other individual treatments (Ayanian and Epstein 1991; Steingart *et al.* 1991; Ayanian *et al.* 1993). Surveys of the public have explored hypothetical 'trade-offs' such as life-saving technologies vs services for people with mental illness (Bowling *et al.* 1993); withholding of life-prolonging medical care from critically ill older persons (Zweibel *et al.* 1993); equity vs cost-effectiveness or good outcomes (Nord *et al.* 1995; Ubel *et al.* 1996); 'do-no-harm' principle vs maximizing outcomes (Baron 1995); helping the worst-off enough vs maximizing outcomes (Ubel and Loewenstein 1995); and personal treatment preferences versus abstract measures of utility (Ubel *et al.* 1996).

The limitation of this body of research is its reliance on quantitative measures, that require the investigator to pre-specify variables of interest (e.g. 'age', 'equity'). This frames the inquiry rigidly, and does not allow deeper insights into inherently complex issues, which are not as neat and discrete in reality as they appear on a survey instrument. For example, representing priority setting as a trade-off between equity and maximizing outcomes oversimplifies the multiplicity of factors involved in these decisions.

Other researchers have employed qualitative research methods to delve into the complexity of priority setting (Crawshaw *et al.* 1985; Dixon and Welch 1991; Klevit *et al.* 1991; Elster 1992; Campbell 1995; Stronks *et al.* 1997). This body of research has successfully uncovered the 'messiness' of priority setting, but because of the reliance on simulation and role-playing, it has revealed little about how people make decisions with real consequences.

Any theory of priority setting that is not empirically grounded may not make sense to those it concerns, and consequently interventions generated from such a theory may be impractical. Moreover, the lack of an empirically grounded conceptual model (i.e. theory) may make it more difficult for different groups (or even the same group) of priority-setting decision makers to make consistent decisions.

Researchers could use a combination of two qualitative methods – grounded theory analysis in the context of case study research – to develop results in the form of an empirically grounded but more generalizable conceptual model. Case study research is 'an empirical inquiry that investigates a contemporary phenomenon within its real-life context, especially when the boundaries between phenomenon and context are not clearly evident' (Yin 1994: 13). Case study research of priority setting could allow analysts to explore both what the real-life decisions are and how real-life decision makers struggle to make them. One fine recent example is a report by Daniels and Sabin (1998a) which explored processes for allocation decisions used by managed care organizations in the USA. Future research could take this approach one step further using grounded theory

methods. Grounded theory is 'a general methodology for developing theory that is grounded in data systematically gathered and
analysed' (Strauss and Corbin 1994: 273). The product would be a
'theory', model, or conceptual framework describing how priority-
setting decisions regarding health technologies are taken in practice.

Connections among discipline-specific perspectives

As noted above, each discipline has its own theoretical approach to
priority setting, but the relationship among these different approaches is often unclear. For example, EBM and CEA approach
priority setting by prioritizing the values of effectiveness and
efficiency. However, these are not the only important values in
priority-setting decisions. This can be confusing to decision makers
and leads to certain 'unsolved rationing problems' (Daniels 1994;
Daniels and Sabin 1997; Singer 1997), outlined below. The extent to
which these problems arise in actual priority-setting contexts, how
they arise, and how they are addressed is not well described.

The fair chances/best outcomes problem

How much should we favour producing the best outcome with our
limited resources (Daniels 1994)? Some philosophers argue that
claims of patients with different probable outcomes should be
equal; some argue that they should be proportional to the differences in outcome; and some that the resource should be allocated
to those with best outcomes.

The priorities problem

How much priority should we give to treating the sickest or most
disabled patients (Daniels 1994)? This problem concerns the 'rule
of rescue' – the perceived duty to save endangered life whenever
possible (Hadorn 1991). For example, our society invests tremendous resources into 'rescuing' people trapped for weeks in
collapsed buildings or 'saving' critically ill patients who have extra-
ordinarily slim chances of survival.

The aggregation problem

When should we allow an aggregation of modest benefits to larger
numbers of people to outweigh more significant benefits to fewer

people? An example of this problem arose in Oregon when tooth capping was prioritized over appendectomy (Daniels 1994). This has been formulated by Kamm as the 'principle of irrelevant utility': 'No number of cured sore throats outweighs saving a life' (Kamm 1994).

The democracy problem

When must we rely on a fair democratic process as the only way to determine what constitutes a fair rationing outcome (Daniels 1994)? Different groups in society have different interests and values, and political processes are important in resource allocation decisions (Bailey 1994). Health care reformers have been experimenting with diverse principles and methods for involving 'community values' in resource allocation decisions, e.g. survey research, 'town-hall' public consultations, *ad hoc* committees with diverse stakeholder representation, as well as democratic, consensus, or elite/expert decision-making models (e.g. Klein 1993b; Lomas 1997a).

The legitimacy problem

Priority setting often means limiting access to health technologies that practitioners and patients may consider either useful or helpful. Under what conditions may such morally controversial decisions be viewed as legitimate, especially to those who disagree (Daniels and Sabin 1997)?

The evidence problem

Information on crucial issues such as treatment effectiveness is often missing, biased, or of poor quality. As a result, the quality of evidence must be balanced against other principles in the decision-making process. For example, should one preferentially fund a programme where there is high-quality evidence of a small benefit, or one where there is lower quality evidence of a large benefit (Singer 1997)?

These unsolved problems highlight shortcomings in the present state of theoretical knowledge related to priority setting. Discipline-specific theories often conflict with other theories from their own or other disciplines and, consequently, are of limited use in solving many problems that commonly arise in priority setting. An interdisciplinary approach may help to reconcile the multiplicity of values that are inherent, and often inherently conflicting, in different discipline-specific perspectives on priority setting (Kahn 1993). Rosenfield (1992) defines interdisciplinary research as 'researchers work[ing] jointly but still from disciplinary-specific basis to address common problem', and transdisciplinary research as 'researchers work[ing] jointly using a shared conceptual framework drawing together disciplinary-specific theories, concepts, and approaches to address common problems'. An interdisciplinary (or transdisciplinary) method, involving scholars from philosophy, law, political science, medicine, economics and other relevant disciplines, can help develop connections between discipline-specific theories, and possibly lead to a shared conceptual framework that transcends traditional disciplinary boundaries.

BEYOND EVIDENCE-BASED MEDICINE AND COST-EFFECTIVENESS ANALYSIS

If you are the medical director in our hypothetical scenario, the prevailing conceptual frameworks of EBM and CEA are helpful tools for determining how your $11 million budget for new technology should be allocated. However, they do not sufficiently account for many of the real considerations that influence decisions in practice, or important theoretical concepts that should influence such decisions.

According to Holm (1998), priority setting has evolved in two phases. The first phase involved a search for 'simple solutions' for rational priority setting (one result of which is the current framework of EBM and CEA). In the second phase, analysts have come to realize that simple solutions are 'theoretically flawed and practically impossible to implement' (Holm 1998: 1002), and attention has focused on the priority-setting process itself (Daniels and Sabin 1997; 1998a; Holm 1998).

The current state of priority setting can be conceptualized as a set of dialectical opposites. For instance, on one axis, substantive criteria for priority setting such as those of cost-effectiveness analysis can be contrasted to process criteria such as those recently developed by Daniels and Sabin in their study of US managed care organizations (Daniels and Sabin 1998b). On another axis, 'simple solutions' (Holm 1998) can be contrasted with 'muddling through', an experimental and incremental process that 'may represent a more sophisticated as well as a more realistic form of rationality than attempts to devise technical fixes' (Klein 1998: 960).

The third phase of priority setting may involve a synthesis that integrates these dialectical opposites. What is needed to advance to the third phase of priority setting is to develop a conceptual framework or model incorporating both substantive and process criteria, and encompassing both 'simple solutions' and 'muddling through'. Such a model must be based in real experience and integrate various theoretical perspectives. How shall this be done? We believe a combination of the case study/grounded theory and interdisciplinary methods described earlier in this chapter may provide the methodology to advance to the third phase of priority setting.

We are currently engaged in developing an empirically grounded, interdisciplinary conceptual model or framework through case studies of priority setting in two meso-level institutions concerned with health technology assessment: Cancer Care Ontario and Cardiac Care Network of Ontario. (The Cancer Care Ontario case actually began with the scenario described at the beginning of this chapter.) Our preliminary results, which were presented at the Second International Conference on Priorities in Health Care, show that a three-facet model (structure, process, outcome) can be used to describe priority setting for new and emerging technologies in these two organizations. The structural facet includes the particulars of the relevant institutions, their mission and mandate, accountability and legitimacy. The process facet includes the people involved in priority setting, relevant information and arguments, transparency, and mechanisms for participation including agenda setting and appeals. The outcomes facet includes the acceptable reasons for decisions and the communication of those decisions. This three-facet model results from a preliminary grounded theory analysis of the two case studies. We have yet to move to the step of interdisciplinary research to make connections between these empirical observations and the discipline-specific theoretical perspectives (and among the discipline-specific perspectives themselves). Nonetheless, for the purpose of this chapter, the three-facet model of priority setting for new and emerging technologies serves as a concrete illustration of how the dialectical opposites of substantive/process criteria and 'simple solutions'/'muddling through' can be synthesized into a conceptual model or framework – representing the third phase of priority setting – using the research method described herein.

Of course, a conceptual model or framework of priority setting derived in the context of health technology assessment will not be completely generalizable to other priority-setting contexts. These other contexts include government decision making (across different social programmes or different envelopes in the health budget), regional health authority decisions (across different health sectors), hospital budget setting (across different hospital programmes), or hospital programme decisions (across different specific services). Although the methodology described herein could be used to study these difference contexts, each of these contexts will need to be studied to elicit important contextual differences. Differences will emerge; for instance, programme quality may be a crucial factor in hospital budget-setting decisions (Singer and Mapa 1998). However, it is also likely that some of the core concepts will be generalizable across contexts (e.g. the legitimacy of the institutions or the people involved in the decision making). Thus, generalizability is best viewed not as an all-or-none concept, but rather as a matter of degree. By studying different contexts, using the same methodology, a generalizable 'theory' (or set of 'theories') of priority setting can ultimately be developed.

In conclusion, the prevailing model of priority setting in health technology assessment is evidence-based medicine and cost-effectiveness analysis. This model is necessary but insufficient to account for both the complexities encountered by decision makers in practice and the conflicting values that different disciplines contribute to thinking about priority setting. 'Simple solutions' on one hand and 'muddling through' on the other, or substantive vs procedural criteria, represent dialectically opposite extremes. A synthesized conceptual model or framework, grounded in real experience and taking account of various discipline-specific perspectives, may represent the third phase of priority setting. Such a model or framework can be developed using the qualitative/inter-disciplinary methodology described herein. As guidelines, or points to consider, the model could provide guidance to decision makers engaged in priority setting for health technology assessment.

ACKNOWLEDGEMENTS

We are grateful to Bernard Dickens, Mita Giacomini and Laura Purdy for participation in an earlier grant proposal on which some of this chapter is based. This research project was supported by grants from the Medical Research Council of Canada (#MA–14675) and the Physicians' Services Incorporated Foundation of Ontario (#98–08).

14

THE RATIONING OF SURGERY: CLINICAL JUDGEMENT VS PRIORITY ACCESS SCORING

Elizabeth Dennett and Bryan Parry

Within the last ten years the New Zealand public health system has undergone a number of reforms. One of the objectives of these reforms was the establishment of the Core Services Committee to define 'core services' or what should be funded in the public health sector. When this task failed it was recommended that specific methods should be developed for prioritizing patients, effectively to ration available resources in a transparent and equitable manner. This led to the development of priority access criteria or methods to calculate a score for patients to determine their priority for elective surgery. Disease-specific priority access criteria were developed on a national basis for cataract surgery, hip and knee joint replacement, transurethral prostatectomy, coronary artery bypass surgery and elective cholecystectomy.

Throughout the reforms the long waiting lists for elective surgery have been an ongoing and contentious issue. Therefore as well as the use of priority access criteria, a booking system has been proposed. To facilitate the introduction of the booking system the use of priority access criteria is to become compulsory (*Sunday Star Times* 1997) and a waiting time fund ($235million) has been established. Access to the waiting time fund was to be based on whether hospitals had:

- priority access criteria in place;
- identified a threshold, that is, a cut-off score for access that is affordable in terms of the anticipated future funding levels; and
- established booking systems to offer some people certainty about when they would receive their surgery (National Advisory Committee 1996).

Though there are five disease-specific priority access criteria available, for general surgery a generic priority access criteria instrument, 'Surgical Priority Criteria Version 2d' (generic SPC), was developed by North Health, the Northern Division of the Transitional Health Authority (now the New Zealand Health Funding Authority) and introduced into Auckland Hospital.

Auckland Hospital is a large teaching hospital of 560 beds, which is staffed by eight general surgeons, four advanced training registrars and four basic training registrars. Every surgeon placing a patient on the waiting list has to complete the generic SPC. The generic SPC requests patient name and diagnosis and is further divided into two sections (Table 14.1), clinical severity (three questions) and total capacity to benefit (two questions). The scores for these two sections are multiplied to give each patient a total out of 100.

The introduction of a generic SPC is understandable in view of the diversity of surgical diagnoses which would otherwise require multiple separate specific priority criteria. Another advantage is that it does not require the determination of relativities between different diagnostic categories. These theoretical advantages notwithstanding, when the generic SPC was introduced in June 1997 no information was provided as to how it had been developed or validated. There was also no request for clinical comment or modification either prior to, or after, its introduction and this led to understandable concern being expressed by clinicians about the clinical applicability and validity of the generic SPC.

We therefore decided to study the likely clinical effectiveness and equity of the generic SPC instrument by comparing the SPC scores for patients on general surgical waiting lists with those obtained using a linear analogue scoring system (LAS). The LAS was designed to quantify the surgeon's assessment of the patient's need for surgery and relative priority.

We then compared three different methods of prioritizing patients for elective cholecystectomy: the regionally developed

Table 14.1   Surgical priority criteria version 2d (generic SPC)

1 *Suffering (physical or mental)*	*Indicative*	*Score*
Mild – occasional and low grade	1	
Moderate – intermittent or low grade	3	
Severe – frequent, inc. night-time, or severe	5	
Incapacitating – dominates life	7	maximum 7
2 *Disability*		
Normal activities difficult	1	
Activities curtailed	3	
Unable to fulfil work/family role	5	
Unable to care for self	7	maximum 7
3 *Clinical cost of delay*		
Poorer outcome following procedure	1	
Progression to more major intervention	3	
High possibility of avoidable disability, illness or death	6	maximum 6
A. *Clinical severity* (add scores 1, 2 & 3)		maximum 20
4 *Degree of improvement anticipated*		
Slight reduction in suffering/disability	0	
Moderate reduction in suffering/disability	1	
Major reduction in suffering/disability	2	maximum 20
5 *Likelihood of improvement*		
25–50% gain significant improvement	1	
50–90% gain significant improvement	2	
>90% gain significant improvement	3	maximum 3
B. *Total capacity to benefit* (add scores 4 & 5)		maximum 5
Total score (multiply A x B) *(clinical severity x total capacity to benefit)*		maximum 100

generic SPC, the nationally developed disease-specific priority access criteria (specific SPC) and the LAS.

STUDY METHODS

From June 1997, data gathered from all new patients on the general surgical waiting lists at Auckland Hospital was collected prospectively. This included a completed generic SPC form, a linear analogue scale (LAS) score and, for those awaiting cholecystectomy, the specific SPC form.

The LAS consisted of a dimensionless line measuring 100mm,

ranging from 'offer operation if no resource constraints' on the left to 'prompt operation essential' on the right. The surgeons and the registrars were asked to place a cross on the LAS where they felt each patient was appropriately situated. The LAS was scored independently of the generic SPC. The surgeons were not blinded to the SPC results of their patients, but they were blinded to the scores that the others gave for the same diagnosis. After two months the data were analysed. The LAS was digitized to a 100-point scale and the mark was converted to a score between 0 and 100.

The data were collected for five months for those requiring cholecystectomy. The specific SPC method, developed by a series of consensus meetings involving selected surgeons and facilitated by the Core Services Committee of the Ministry of Health, consists of seven questions (Table 14.2), the answers to which are scored. The scores are then added together to give a total score (maximum 100).

Since the data were not normally distributed, non-parametric tests were used for statistical analysis. Correlation coefficients were calculated using the Spearman rank correlation coefficient, and the Mann-Whitney U test was used to check differences in mean values. The limits of agreement analysis was performed as described by Bland and Altman (1986). When two methods of measurement (here, the SPC and the LAS) are compared neither provides an unequivocally correct answer. By using simple calculations (the average of the two scores for each patient and the difference between the two scores for each patient) a limits of agreement analysis determines the degree of agreement between the two methods. Perfect agreement between two methods of measurement would produce a numerical result of zero.

RESULTS

A total of 230 generic SPC forms were completed, 21(9%) being rejected for analysis due to incomplete information or illegibility. Of the other 209, 59 had a diagnosis of cancer, the majority being breast (21) and colorectal (20). The 150 generic SPC forms with a benign diagnosis were spread across many diagnostic groups, with hernia being the most numerous (42).

The distribution of generic SPC and LAS scores for all diagnoses have been plotted as frequency histograms (Figure 14.1). The median (range) for the generic SPC and LAS were 35 (10–100) and 80 (0–100) respectively, p < 0.0001. There was a clear difference

Table 14.2   Priority criteria for elective cholecystectomy (specific SPC)

Frequency of biliary-type pain	
3 or more attacks/past month	15
1–2 attacks past month	10
3 or more attacks/past year	5
1–2 attacks/past year	2
Average severity of biliary-type pain[1]	
Severe	15
Mild–moderate	5
Average duration of attack of biliary-type pain	
>6 hours	15
1–6 hours	10
<1 hour	5
Disturbance in patient's life due to symptoms	
Major disturbance	20
Minor disturbance	10
None	0
History of acute cholecystitis (single episode)[2]	
Yes	15
No	0
Past history of common bile duct stones[3]	
Without subsequent demonstration of duct clearance (e.g. jaundice, cholangitis, gallstone pancreatitis)	15
With subsequent demonstration of duct clearance	5
Presence of diabetes	
Yes	5
No	0

Notes:
[1] 'Severe' means that intramuscular narcotics are required; 'mild–moderate' means that oral agents are sufficient to alleviate pain
[2] A second episode of acute cholecystitis warrants immediate intervention and these criteria do not apply
[3] Clinical evidence of current common bile duct stone warrants immediate intervention and these criteria do not apply

between the two scoring systems with the generic SPC dominated by low scores, 50 per cent being less than 40; by contrast the LAS had predominantly high scores with more than 50 per cent being greater than 70.

The distribution of the generic SPC and LAS scores excluding

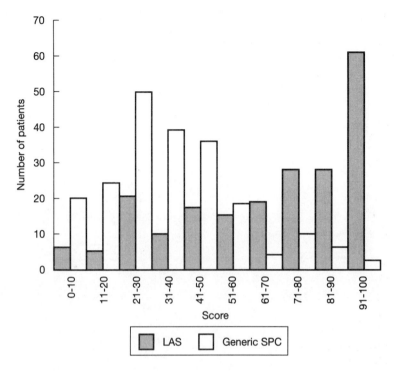

Figure 14.1 Frequency distribution for the generic SPC and LAS

Source: Dennett 1998a (reproduced with permission)

the cancers are shown in Figure 14.2. In this case the medians (ranges) were 33 (10–100) and 65 (0–100) respectively, p < 0.0001, and there were similar though less pronounced differences.

The correlation coefficients and limits of agreement analysis are summarized in Table 14.3. Overall there was a striking difference in correlation coefficients and range of scores between the cancer and benign subgroups.

Although the correlation coefficient for all data was 0.464 (p < 0.0001), the limits of agreement analysis demonstrated little agreement between the two. The potential difference in scores between the SPC and the LAS for each patient was 50 points.

The scores given by six of the surgeons were also compared. The median score given for all patients using the generic SPC varied widely, ranging from 22.9 to 45.7 (p < 0.0001). There was no

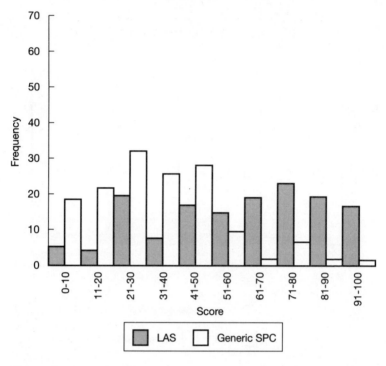

Figure 14.2   Frequency histogram for the generic SPC and LAS minus the cancer diagnoses

Source: Dennett 1998a (reproduced with permission)

significant difference in the scores given using the LAS (range 60.2 to 74.9). This wide spread of median generic SPC scores was also seen when the results were further divided into diagnostic groups, e.g. cancer (32.4 to 70.7, p = 0.003) and hernia (14.6 to 36.6, p = 0.003). Again there was no significant difference in the scores given using the LAS, cancer (96.5 to 100, p = 0.9118) and hernia (32.1 to 58.9, p = 0.336).

For cholecystectomy, a total of 22 patients were scored by three surgeons and four registrars using the three methods. The scores from the specific SPC (median 45, range 15 to 80) had a bimodal distribution. The scores from the generic SPC (median 26, range 3 to 80) were negatively skewed and the LAS scores (median 70, range 30 to 100) were positively skewed (Figure 14.3).

Table 14.3 Correlation coefficient (Spearman), mean difference and 95% confidence intervals for limits of agreement analysis

Category	n	Correlation coefficient	p value	Mean difference in score	95% confidence interval
All data	209	0.46	<0.0001	33.3	–17.7–84.4
All benign	150	0.52	<0.0001	27.0	–21.0–75.0
Hernia	42	0.57	0.0003	13.6	–33.2–60.5
Gastrointestinal	55	0.54	<0.0001	31.7	–11.9–75.2
Anorectal	29	0.55	0.0036	34.6	–10.6–79.8
All cancer	59	0.09	0.481	49.8	41.4–91.2
Breast cancer	21	0.08	0.718	52.3	12.7–92.0
Colorectal cancer	20	0.10	0.651	52.0	6.4–97.6
Other cancer	18	0.38	0.114	44.3	–7.5–96.0

Source: Dennett 1998a (reproduced with permission)

There were significant positive correlations between the scores of the specific and generic SPCs ($r = 0.69$, $p = 0.002$) and the specific SPC and LAS ($r = 0.61$, $p = 0.005$), but not between the generic SPC and LAS ($r = 0.41$, $p = 0.059$).

The results of the limits of agreement analysis for the three cholecystectomy scoring methods showed that, for any individual, there could be an average difference of ± 36 points between the three. This meant, for example, if a patient scored 60 with the specific SPC they could score anywhere from 24 to 96 points with the generic SPC and LAS.

DISCUSSION

Problems arose during the development of the previous standardized assessment criteria, particularly that for cholecystectomy. A number of the clinicians involved felt it was a pointless exercise, so consensus was difficult to achieve. Furthermore, the clinicians were concerned that arbitrary cut-off points would be created below which surgery would not be funded though they were told this would not happen. Hadorn and Holmes (1997) suggest these criteria can be used as a means of deciding which patients will or will not receive surgery under various possible levels of funding. This

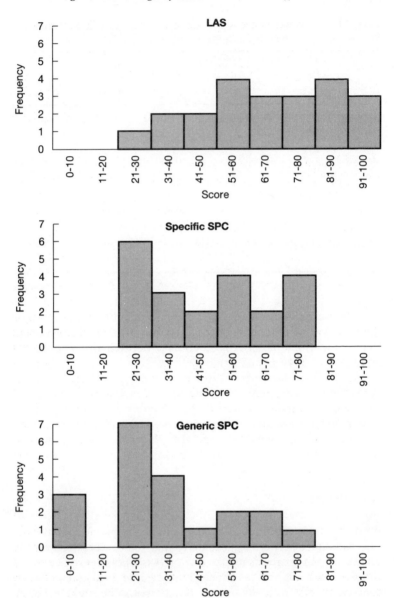

Figure 14.3   Frequency distribution of total scores for the three scoring methods

Source: Dennett 1998b (reproduced with permission)

highlights the need to develop tools which have credibility with the clinicians and to ensure that they are accurate and reproducible.

One of the concerns of the general surgeons in the Auckland Hospital was that no attempt had been made to identify the criteria used by clinicians in normal clinical practice to determine expected benefit. We have shown that correlation between the LAS and the generic SPC was poor and there was little consistency between the surgeons in the scores allocated for the same diagnosis. The limits of agreement are so wide they cannot be applied reliably to individual patients. During the development of the criteria for laparoscopic cholecystectomy, the weighting given to the presence of diabetes or history of acute cholecystitis was in the opposite direction to the expectations of the developers, despite the clinical importance of these factors (New Zealand Core Services Committee 1995).

The difference between the generic SPC and the judgements of expert clinicians (LAS) is best exemplified by those patients with a diagnosis of cancer. The New Zealand Ministry of Health reported (*New Zealand Herald* 1997) that use of these priority criteria would remove 34 per cent of patients from the waiting lists. This would mean adopting a threshold score of 25 points on the generic SPC for general surgery. If the SPC was strictly applied 20 per cent of patients with any diagnosis of cancer would have to be removed from the waiting lists. It is widely expected that further funding cuts will require waiting list reductions of 50 per cent. This would mean the SPC threshold would have to be raised to 35 points and 41 per cent of cancer patients would not get their surgery. If the LAS was used instead, the threshold would be 80 but 95 per cent of cancer patients would still get their surgery. The generic SPC does not enable you to take account of the diagnosis in this way and cancer patients consistently score lower than patients with benign diagnoses.

The under-responsiveness to malignancy is probably caused by the question on 'clinical cost of delay' which fails to distinguish between delay leading to disability, illness or death. Consequently both benign and malignant conditions are equally likely to score the maximum six points. This 'coarseness' of measurement is also a problem with Questions 4 and 5 (Table 14.1). The degree of anticipated improvement or likelihood of improvement should be different for benign and malignant conditions.

This type of comparison between holistic scores like the LAS and scores derived from instruments such as the generic SPC needs to be treated with caution. Linear analogue scales provide an efficient method of summarizing information in a way that is amenable to measurement and have been extensively used in surgical research, for example to measure pain or fatigue. The advantages of such a technique are that it is easy to grasp; it is quick to fill out and score; it does not require much motivation on the part of the patient; and, as surgeons are not restricted to direct quantitative terms, they can make as fine a discrimination as they wish (Bond and Lader 1974). Our study did not attempt to validate the LAS formally, but it is striking that there was consistency in the median scores for the LAS given by a randomly selected group of surgeons. Taking previous work into consideration we consider it a fair and convenient summary of expert clinical judgement.

The original five disease-specific priority criteria already developed are examples of multiple factor additive systems known as linear models (Dawes and Corrigan 1974). With these, each question asked has a range of acceptable answers, each with its own score. The individual scores are added together to give a total score, usually out of a maximum of 100. The priority criteria for elective cholecystectomy (Table 14.2) is an example of this. The generic SPC, however, uses a multiplication ingredient. The sum of the scores for Questions 1–3 is multiplied by the sum of the scores for Questions 4 and 5, to give a total out of 100. This results, not surprisingly, in poor diagnostic discrimination as all patients, whatever the diagnosis, obtain a score within a very narrow range.

As there was no relationship between scores on the generic SPC and the LAS, the elective cholecystectomy study was undertaken to see if the disease-specific priority access criteria performed better, that is more consistently with the LAS scores. As with the generic SPC, the specific SPC for elective cholecystectomy bore little relation to clinical judgement as determined by the dissimilar distribution of the scores the patients obtained.

The distribution of scores for all three methods was different. The LAS was positively skewed because the clinicians tended to feel that treatment was warranted because patients had symptoms. The generic SPC was negatively skewed, consistent with its origin as a tool introduced by a funding body for rationing purposes. Interestingly, the specific SPC had a bimodal distribution which may be closer to clinical reality, the lower peak representing those patients who were considered appropriate candidates for elective surgery and the upper peak those who were felt to need surgery urgently.

In assessing the relationship between the methods it is perhaps not coincidental that the specific SPC method, which was developed in conjunction with clinicians, produced scores closer to those obtained by the LAS than the generic SPC. In spite of this, there is little agreement between any of the scoring methods, as shown by the ±30-point difference between scores for any individual patient.

These results suggest that the newer 'objective' methods represent no advance on clinical judgement; indeed they appear considerably worse. It is not clear whether this whole approach to rationing health services is fundamentally flawed or whether the optimal scoring method has yet to be devised. If better scoring systems are to be produced, it will be important to base them on sound evidence and to develop them in collaboration with clinicians, epidemiologists and the general public.

In 1993 the National Health Advisory Committee on Health and Disability issued a consultation document called *Seeking Consensus*. From this inadequate consultation the committee took the view that 'the public' accepted the principle of treating people on the basis of likely benefit, using priority assessment criteria (Holmes and Smith 1997).

Unlike the approaches to priority setting adopted in Oregon (Bodenheimer 1997) and Sweden (Swedish Parliamentary Priorities Commission 1995), the New Zealand priority access criteria determine funding on the basis of the patient rather than the procedure. The Oregon Health Plan was developed because of the escalating cost of Medicaid cover. In exchange for increasing the number of people eligible for Medicaid, fewer services would be provided. After three years of work involving consultation with the public and health service providers, more than 700 diagnoses and treatments were ranked in order of importance. The state legislature then drew a cut-off line; treatments below the line would not be covered by Medicaid. The system suffers from the two problems common to the establishment of priority criteria. The first problem is 'gaming', which is where doctors select a diagnosis above the threshold or decide on a score and then complete the form in such a way as to ensure the patient exceeds the threshold. The second problem is the arbitrary movement of the threshold. For example, in two years the Oregon state legislature has moved the threshold and reduced the number of procedures funded. The New Zealand priority access initiatives have not begun to address these two problems.

In New Zealand a modified Delphi technique (Hadorn and Holmes 1997) was used to develop the specific priority access criteria. This technique enables a large group of experts to be contacted at minimal cost, but it is vulnerable to poor questionnaire design and inadequate testing of reliability, and it can force consensus rather than allowing discussion to occur (Jones and Hunter 1995). In contrast, the generic SPC was an initiative from a funding authority and reflects an emphasis on cost containment. There was no formal input from clinicians or the community in its formulation. Another problem with both these 'objective' methods is that they involve a significant subjective element because of the need to interpret individual questions which lack clear definition.

One of the potential problems with this study was the way the scoring was undertaken. The generic SPC was usually completed first, followed by LAS, and for the cholecystectomy patients the specific SPC was usually completed between the generic SPC and LAS. Randomization of the order would have minimized any influence the first score had on any subsequent scores. The tools used (generic SPC; cholecystectomy-specific SPC) would have been strengthened if inter-observer reliability had been determined first. This, along with validity, is something that should have been established by those who developed the methods before they were introduced. This study goes some way towards identifying the problems that have occurred because this was not done. Rather than a weakness of the study the relatively large number of observers approximates the real clinical context in which these tools are to be applied. Recently it has been demonstrated that increasing the number of data points and varying the number of observers did not alter the extent of the variation between the scoring (Dennett and Parry 1998).

The fundamental issue that should be addressed before introducing priority access criteria is to determine the scope of public health care provision. This was the original task of the Core Services Committee. Until we have decided what procedures should be funded in the public sector, any initiative to determine whether an individual patient should or should not receive a particular procedure is meaningless. The question of the threshold for access to care is an important public issue. Wide consultation among the general public, health care professionals and government representatives is still required to address these issues. Priority access criteria developed as a result of this process should be tested to demonstrate that they are valid, repeatable, generalizable, and not susceptible to gaming. Scoring systems should be introduced in such a way that clinicians understand the basis and objectives of the initiative.

The most definitive evidence we could acquire about the validity of priority access criteria would be to see if patients are harmed as a result of being removed from waiting lists following use of these tools. A repeat of our study with follow-up to look at clinical outcomes would answer this question. Our study suggests much work remains to be done.

ACKNOWLEDGEMENTS

Professor G. Hill for the original suggestion of the LAS and Dr L. Plank for invaluable statistical help, both from the Department of Surgery, University of Auckland.

PART VI

INVOLVING THE PUBLIC

explicat?

15

PUBLIC INVOLVEMENT IN HEALTH CARE PRIORITY SETTING: ARE THE METHODS APPROPRIATE AND VALID?

Penelope M. Mullen

There is increasing interest in involving the public in priority setting in the UK and elsewhere. However, there is evidence of lack of clarity in the objectives of some priority-setting projects and about the role of public involvement.[1] Further, some projects display an apparent ignorance of both long-standing theoretical literature and practical experience of methods for deriving priorities in health care and related fields.

PUBLIC INVOLVEMENT

Although many commentators appear to consider its desirability as axiomatic, the notion of public involvement in health care priority setting is not unproblematic.[2] For instance, Grimley Evans (1993: 50) argues that an approach that puts the rights of individual citizens in the hands of other citizens is fallacious as 'one of the principles of the British state is that all citizens are equal in having equal status before the law and equal basic access to the means of life, education and health'.

Concerns about the legitimacy of public involvement relate to the 'representativeness' of those participating, the perceived lack of knowledge of lay people in an area populated by professionals, the risk of populism and even public resistance to being involved in 'rationing'. There is also concern that public participation is being used to compensate for the lack of democracy – the democratic deficit – in the UK, since members of health authorities are appointed, not elected. Thus, interest in public involvement within the NHS could be viewed either as an attempt to compensate for the lack of elected democratic control or as an attempt to distract attention from the lack of such control (Pollock 1992).

Involving the public in priority setting can serve to legitimize the resulting decisions, seen as an advantage by Ham (1993) but viewed with concern by Hunter (1993). This leads to Fleck's (1994: 375) prior consent argument where he states that 'if all who will be affected by rationing decisions have a fair opportunity to shape these decisions, then these rationing decisions will be freely self-imposed, which is an essential feature of just rationing decisions'. But can a majority view of the public be taken to imply prior consent by all members to restrictions on services or treatments?

The extent and type of public involvement in health care vary considerably (Feuerstein 1980). Arnstein (1969) demonstrated this in her useful 'ladder of participation', which descends from citizen control, through consultation and informing, to manipulation. Mullen *et al.* (1984) made a distinction between 'reactive' and 'pro-active' or 'initiator' involvement. Such distinctions affect not only approaches to involvement but also how the function, validity and very nature of public involvement are viewed by health care providers and by society.

PRIORITY SETTING

The spectre of 'rationing' overshadows priority setting: indeed many consider the terms synonymous. There appears to be a widespread assumption that rationing is inevitable with the only questions being how it should be done, how explicitly, and what role the public should play. However, the 'inevitability' of rationing has been challenged (Mullen 1998a *inter alia*) and its unquestioning acceptance may distort priority-setting projects involving the public by focusing on denial, stressing the need for 'hard choices' and detracting from the many other areas where choices must be made in delivering health care services and where priority setting is essential. In addition, rationing raises a number of issues, discussed elsewhere (Mullen 1998b), which have implications for public involvement.

Nevertheless, priorities are set and choices are made in many different contexts. At government level, priorities are set between the NHS and competing claims for funds; NHS resources are allocated between geographical areas and specialties; choices are made between centralizing and dispersing facilities; priorities involve the order and the way in which services are delivered (e.g. what priority to give to the right to choose a female doctor); and decisions are made between individual patients.

These raise a number of opportunities and areas for public involvement:

- ethos/values of the NHS
  (e.g. rights to health care);
- what health care services/treatments are provided
  (scope of NHS);
- which groups should receive priority
  (e.g. old vs young; employed vs unemployed);
- location of health service provision
  (e.g. locally vs centrally; institution vs community);
- non-medical aspects
  (e.g. appointment systems; waiting; food; decor);
- choice of treatment for individual patient
  (individual involvement; empowerment).

Many of the controversial, and even exciting, debates centre around the second and third areas. However, in practice, public involvement frequently focuses on the fourth and fifth. These relate to *how* services are provided and are of considerable importance to providers and users of health services. They offer considerable scope for public involvement and few problems of legitimacy but have been overshadowed in recent debates by questions of which services should be provided and to whom – explicit rationing.

LOCAL VS NATIONAL

Clearly, even within a *national* health service, equity does not require identical services everywhere. Indeed, differential needs, because of demography, epidemiology and topology etc., require inter-locality differences in services in order to achieve equity. However, is it legitimate, within a national health service, for local priority setting, even with public involvement, to result in people with identical health care needs and in identical circumstances having different access to services solely because of where they live?

APPROACHES TO 'ENGAGING' THE PUBLIC

The objectives of the exercise – the use to which the results will be put and the type of priority setting being addressed – will determine who should be involved (the target population), and how. The target population may consist of the general population at large, users of a specific service or sufferers from a particular condition. The choice of methodology to 'engage' the public will also be influenced by whether the aim is to obtain results generalizable to the whole target population or to 'set the agenda', e.g. determine which issues are of concern to respondents.

A wide range of methods are used to involve the public. Some 'mass' approaches, such as telephone hotlines, public meetings, advertisements in newspapers and leaflets, sometimes including reply forms or simple questionnaires, largely leave the initiative to the public to become involved. Other 'mass' approaches include large-scale, statistically valid surveys, using either self-completion questionnaires or interviews.

Of increasing popularity, especially to identify issues of concern to users or the public, are small-scale discussion or focus groups. Some such groups are constructed to be 'representative' of their target population, while the make-up of others is more opportunistic.

Some approaches use proxies. One method attempts to determine patients' views by surveying GPs, despite evidence that GPs' views can differ considerably from those of their patients (Bowling *et al.* 1993, *inter alia*). Rapid Appraisal, pioneered in developing countries, is increasingly popular. This seeks to determine community views by interviewing key people (e.g. teachers, home helps, corner-shop owners etc.) deemed to be in touch with local opinion.

Some methodologies attempt to ensure 'informed' involvement by providing participants with information. Citizens' Juries, where a 'representative' panel of 'citizens' meet over several days, hear evidence on a particular issue and 'deliver their verdict' (Stewart *et al.* 1994; Leneghan *et al.* 1996; Dunkerley and Glasner 1998). 'Standing' groups of consumers, who are involved over a period of time, have been assembled. These range from focus groups with continuing membership, which meet periodically (Richardson

1997), to standing panels of over 1000 local residents, who complete questionnaires on different issues. However, informing the public prior to their involvement, and repeated involvement of the same members of the public, may not always be appropriate. There may well be instances where the objective is to secure involvement by the public 'at large', 'uncontaminated' by professional views or information.

METHODS OF ELICITING VALUES

There are a number of methods for eliciting values and preferences, either explicitly or implicitly, some of which are listed below:

Single vote
Multiple vote
Ranking
Budget pie
Scoring/rating
Scaling:
  Likert-type scale
  Visual analogue scale
Delphi-type methods
Simple paired comparison
Weighted paired comparison
Constant-sum paired comparison
Scaled paired comparison
Analytical Hierarchy Process
Conjoint Analysis
Measure of Value
Time trade-off
Standard Gamble
Willingness to Pay (WTP)
Qualitative Discriminant Process
Simple trade-off (compensation or sacrifice)
Priority Search
Constrained ranking
Aggregated scores

Such techniques have a long history in many disciplines, including economics, operational research, psychology, political science and philosophy, and many are grounded within those disciplinary theories. However, theoretical validity does not always coincide with acceptability, people's comprehension and even people's value systems. It is thus important to get the correct balance between theoretical validity and user acceptability. At the very least, users should understand the values implicit in their chosen technique, the form of choice being imposed on respondents, the implications of aggregation and, most importantly, its appropriateness for the purpose of the exercise.

Single vs multi-attribute

Most health care decisions are multi-criterion or multi-attribute. Thus some approaches incorporate two or more separate stages, valuing first the attributes/criteria and then evaluating the options against those criteria. However, some, Conjoint Analysis for example (Ryan 1996), infer the attribute values implicitly from choices expressed between options possessing different 'levels' of the various attributes. In practice, single-stage approaches are often used, even when valuing multi-attribute options, such as treatments or packages of care. Other exercises invite the public to value attributes such as access, waiting times, friendliness of staff etc., without explicitly incorporating the resulting values into a two-stage model.

Constrained vs unconstrained

Techniques for eliciting values either require respondents to make constrained (or forced) choices which 'incorporate some notion of sacrifice' (Shackley and Ryan 1995: 198), or allow unconstrained choices or valuations. The latter are characterized by scaling methods, where each criterion/attribute/option is valued independently of the others. Constrained choices involve some form of trade-off between different attributes or alternatives and include a wide range of voting, ranking, comparison and trade-off techniques.

Generally, if the attributes or options being valued are independent and not in competition, unconstrained-choice methods are preferred. For psychological reasons, such methods might also be appropriate where attributes, such as equity and access, are being valued, even if subsequent normalization effectively constrains choices. However, constrained-choice methods are indicated where options are in competition and/or the purpose of the exercise is to introduce respondents to the concept of trade-off or sacrifice. However, if options are mutually exclusive, some constrained-choice methodologies, such as budget pie, do not work. Unconstrained valuations can cause specific problems in aggregation, especially relating to inter-person equity.

Intensity of preference

Generally, permitting respondents to indicate intensity of preference, using methods such as scaling/rating or budget pie (where each respondent is given a fixed 'budget' of points/tokens (often 100) or money to allocate between options in any amounts they choose), is preferred. But where the objective is to force choices between two or more options, indication of intensity of preference may be inappropriate. There are possible dangers with methods, such as single and multiple vote, which force specific 'intensity of preference' values which may not accord with the respondent's values. There are also potential problems with methods which, without the respondent's knowledge, impose implied preference values on their choices, for example using rank positions as 'scores' or assigning 'scores' to responses on a Likert scale.

Money

Methodologies which employ money, such as some variants of budget pie and willingness-to-pay (WTP), can encounter specific problems. The latter can face respondent resistance or under-valuation where WTP is being sought for options which are normally provided free at the point of use, such as items of health care. Further, despite some imaginative attempts (Donaldson 1995), the problem of the effect of respondents' differential purchasing power has not been satisfactorily resolved. In addition, although appearing to be the archetypal constrained method involving 'notions of sacrifice', when WTP is used to value publicly provided services, respondents' choices are constrained only by their own personal disposable income, not by a constrained public budget.

Budget pie and its two-option variant, constant-sum paired comparison (where the 'budget' is divided between two options only), overcome these problems as respondents are allocated a 'budget'. However, the absolute size of that budget raises problems. Realistic sums for health care options are probably outside the normal experience of respondents. Small sums, say £100, risk seeming trivial. Experience suggests budget pie methods work better when respondents are allocated tokens or points rather than money.

However, sufficient tokens (c. 100) should be allocated to permit respondents sufficient discrimination in allocating them between options. One unpublished study, with a budget of only 15 tokens, reported respondents wishing to cut tokens in half.

Aggregation

Aggregation of individual values poses potentially insoluble ethical and theoretical problems. At the simplest ethical level, is it legitimate to combine one person's rating of 10 with another's rating of 0 and conclude that the group or societal rating is 5? The theoretical debate takes us into the field of social welfare and social choice and has generated a vast literature. Arguments range from the impossibility of making inter-personal comparisons of utility, thus arguing that aggregating values across individuals is impermissible, to those who argue that societal choices have to be made – using the example of voting in elections – so we should stop arguing and simply add up the individual values. While the latter argument has some force, the theoretical literature should not be ignored.

Arrow's *Impossibility Theorem*, which, argues Pattanaik (1997: 205), 'is the most celebrated impossibility theorem in the literature on social choice theory', shows that there is no way to aggregate individual choices that satisfies a set of minimum conditions and axioms. These include transitivity (if x is preferred to y and y to z, then x is preferred to z), non-dictatorship (no individual's preferences are imposed as the societal preferences) and the weak Pareto criterion (if all individuals prefer x to y, then society must prefer x to y) (Arrow 1963a). Possibly of greatest interest in the NHS, given the proliferation of ranking exercises, is Arrow's Condition 3 – the Independence of Irrelevant Alternatives. This requires that the preference ordering of a set of alternatives is unaffected by the addition (or subtraction) of an 'irrelevant' alternative, i.e. if A is preferred to B and B is preferred to C, the introduction of an 'irrelevant' alternative D should not alter the ABC ordering, wherever D itself is placed in the ordering. It is easy to demonstrate how this condition can be violated when rank positions are used as scores and summed.

Condorcet's *Voting Paradox* demonstrates that aggregation of transitive preferences of individuals can yield intransitive 'group' preferences; that is, even if each individual has transitive preferences, it is possible, when the individual preferences are aggregated, that the group preferences are intransitive, that is, the group prefers x to y, y to z, but prefers z to x (Brown and Jackson 1978: 72–4; McLean 1987: 26 *inter alia*).

This should not be dismissed simply as theoretical game playing. Ranking is used widely within the NHS for eliciting values with the rank positions frequently being converted to 'scores' and summed. The potential for manipulating results, whether intentionally or inadvertently, by including *irrelevant* options must be recognized. Further, the method of aggregation can affect the result. As Weale (1990: 122) points out, 'The same set of preferences in a community amalgamated by a difference voting rule will yield a different collective choice.'

At the very least, users of techniques should be aware of the dangers of aggregation and of the implications of different methods. Perez (1994), agreeing that there is no truly satisfactory procedure for the aggregation of preferences in ordinal contexts, suggests that a framework should be devised to help choose a relatively good rule for a given situation. In addition, because of the problems associated with aggregation, it is often better to avoid single aggregated measures and present, instead, the full distribution of results, using bar charts or histograms.

Aggregation also raises issues of inter-respondent equity. Several techniques, such as voting and budget pie, give respondents equal weight unless a deliberate choice is made to award unequal numbers of votes or unequal budgets. However, with scoring or rating or where, for instance, rank positions are summed but not all respondents rank the same number of options, respondents may unintentionally acquire unequal weights. This may be desirable in some applications but it is important to prevent accidental inter-respondent inequity.

Ease of use and transparency

While it is desirable that techniques are easy to use for respondents, whether or not such techniques should be transparent – in the sense that respondents can see how their responses are going to be used and how they contribute to the final scores – will depend on the application. While there must be a presumption in favour of transparency, lack of transparency may sometimes be an essential part of the research process. Further, transparency could lead to strategic 'voting'.

Clearly, researchers should understand the techniques used, their implications and, in particular, how the final 'scores' are produced and their interpretation. Dangers can arise especially from the use of computer software, which permits researchers to employ methodologies which they do not fully understand. There is considerable evidence within the NHS that the implications of some of the methodologies employed are not fully understood.

CHOICE OF TECHNIQUE FOR ELICITING VALUES

A major question is how necessary it is to be concerned with the theoretical bases of techniques. Although some researchers argue it is essential that techniques are grounded in the theory of their own discipline, it is proposed here that a more pragmatic stance be adopted. Thus, it is suggested, the questions in Table 15.1 should be asked when considering the appropriateness of techniques for a particular application. An approach which is ideal in one situation may prove totally inappropriate or misleading in another.

Such a pragmatic stance has long-standing support. For instance,

Table 15.1 Questions to be asked of techniques

Appropriateness
- Is the technique appropriate to the problem or issues to which it is to be applied?
- Does it take account of how the problem or issues are likely to be perceived by respondents?
- Are the ways in which respondents are permitted to answer meaningful both to them and to the problem?
- Does the technique seek constrained or unconstrained choices?
- Does the technique permit respondents to indicate intensity of preference?
- How exactly are responses to be interpreted?

Aggregation
- Is the aggregation method appropriate to the situation?
- Is any inter-respondent inequity intentional?

Ease of use
- How easy is the technique for respondents to use?
- How transparent is the technique to the respondents and to users?
- Are its implications generally understood by users?
- Does the technique require skilled staff to administer it?

Huber (1974), demonstrating that different methods of eliciting values are equally good predictors of clients' preferences, concluded that transparency is important and that the major choice criterion should be acceptability of the method to the client. Clark (1974: 26) suggests that 'one good principle is to utilize instruments only as precise and complex as necessary for the decision at hand', adding that 'the instruments can be no more sensitive than their users'. However, the choice of method is not unimportant. In a small-scale study comparing budget pie, which permits expression of intensity of preference, with multiple vote, which does not, Mullen (1983) demonstrated that very different individual and aggregated group values resulted.

CONCLUSION

A large amount of energy and resources appear to be being directed to public involvement but there is evidence of 'reinvention of the wheel' and some lack of awareness of previous work and the range of techniques available both for 'engaging' the public and for eliciting values. Further, few projects exhibit awareness of ethical and technical problems associated with the aggregation of individual values.

But how necessary is it to be concerned about the technical validity of methodologies used? The answer must lie partly in the purpose of such projects. If the public involvement *process* is the prime objective – and there are repeated reports of the benefit gained from the process itself – then methodological validity is of secondary importance. However, if the results are used to determine (or even inform) priorities and resource redeployment, it would appear essential to have regard for methodological validity and to ensure that users understand the implications of the methods employed.

These points were stressed many years ago by Hoinville and Courtenay (1979: 175) who, after ten years of conducting public consultation exercises, concluded that there is no single technique or easy solution. 'Measurements have to be tailored to the application to which they will be put. Questions must be as closely linked as possible to the way the answers will be used.'

NOTES

1 In addition to published sources, this chapter draws on results from a survey of projects on 'Involving the Public in Priority Setting' in UK health authorities carried out with Peter Spurgeon.
2 The focus here is on involvement or participation collectively as 'citizens' and (potential) users, rather than individual patients 'participating' in decisions about their own treatment. However, participation by, say, user groups may cloud this distinction.

16

RATIONING HEALTH CARE IN NEW ZEALAND – HOW THE PUBLIC HAS A SAY

Wendy Edgar

New Zealand's National Health Committee (NHC) was set up in 1992 to advise the government on the types of health and disability services that should be publicly funded and their relative priorities, with due regard to available resources. A key task was to advance the public debate and understanding of the limits on health care resources, and the need to make choices about which services would be funded and for whom.[1] The health purchaser in New Zealand, the Health Funding Authority (HFA) (previously four regional health authorities) is also obliged to consult about its plans for the purchase of services. The public consultation work of the NHC and the HFA have become increasingly complementary over time. The distinction is that the NHC's work in involving the public is at the level of principles, broad service priorities or statements of service effectiveness – as policy advice – and the HFA's consultations are at the implementation level – that is, within the resources HFA has, what services it plans to purchase and where, with what specific access criteria or part charges. This chapter describes the work of the National Health Committee.

ASSUMPTIONS

Four assumptions underlie the NHC's position when consulting with the public:

- Rationing of publicly funded health services is inevitable in New Zealand – irrespective of total levels of funding, it is expected that demand for services will always be greater than can be afforded. Because funding is finite, choices will have to be made about what is funded publicly.

- Decisions about which services are to be funded and who is to get those services must be transparent – arrived at through open discussion, with fair and transparent processes.
- Communities, the general public, must be involved – their values are important for overall service priorities, a fair balance of needs, and acceptable principles and decision processes on who is to receive funded services.
- Best practice guidelines and priority criteria are explicit tools which can help transparent decision making – they are technical devices to assist professionals in making better decisions in the use of resources and, published as consumer pamphlets, can allow the public to be more fully informed.

CLARIFYING TERMS

For the NHC, 'the public' means 'New Zealanders living in communities throughout the country'. But 'the public' is not a simple concept. We are all members of the public. We have all been exposed to the health sector at some stage in our lives – and we almost all have firm views about it. We experience ill health, either personally or through family members, neighbours or friends. As members of a community, we may be health service users, service providers, policy makers, client advocates, or carers of ill or disabled family members. The media, expert commentators, the pharmaceutical industry, groups with moral authority such as the clergy and the judiciary are also part of the public – and are extremely influential in shaping public perceptions.

The point is that health is such a personal and sometimes emotional issue that no one is totally uninvolved or unbiased. The differences lie in the knowledge individuals have. So when the NHC involves the public in project work or goes out to talk to the public in communities, it expects to see a range of people with different levels of understanding, and agendas, in each public audience.

I have deliberately chosen to use the word 'rationing' rather than 'setting priorities' or 'prioritizing'. 'Rationing' often has pejorative connotations, implying for many a reduction in funding and loss of services. The NHC regards the word as more honest and direct than prioritizing or priority setting, however, because it explicitly acknowledges that there is a finite resource, inevitably involving service trade-offs when more emphasis is to be given to services regarded as more important. The context for NHC work was, and still is, to be cognisant of the government's limited resources in advising on services to be publicly funded.[2]

'Consultation' is also a concept with many interpretations. The 'ideal' of inclusive, democratic decision making is probably not achievable, even with a population as small as New Zealand's 3.8 million. However, how each consultation meeting is characterized, the expectations that participants bring to meetings for the outcomes of their involvement, and whether those understandings are clarified, will determine whether the public see involvement as worthwhile or not.

For the NHC, the audience and the purposes of many consultation activities have been multi-layered. Objectives have ranged from information sharing and awareness raising, through opinion gathering, to input on specific questions or identification of service priorities. This reflects, first, the evolving nature of the rationing debate in New Zealand – the NHC is still, six years on, using a variety of approaches with differing purposes and engaging different audiences. Second, striving for 'a public view' on rationing may not be a sensible goal. There will always be many views, depending on the audience and the issue of the day.[3]

IS PUBLIC INVOLVEMENT WORTHWHILE?

Despite the challenges, the NHC believes that the public must be involved. Debating the issues is an ongoing requirement of health rationing. There are no single answers which hold for all time. What is needed is a continuing dialogue – for information, awareness of the complexities, understanding of the principles and decision processes to be used, and engagement at least, if not always acceptance of what is decided.

For the NHC, it becomes not so much an issue of when to consult, but to what extent and with whom. None of the NHC's advice is offered to the Minister of Health without first seeking and sifting through contributions which are sought from outside the committee. Since 1992, a range of methods has been used for involving the public, both face-to-face (such as through town hall meetings, focus groups or consensus conferences) and indirectly (for example through submission processes).

In weighting public contributions, the NHC takes the view that public consultation is one strand among many that make up final decisions on any matter. It has been given the responsibility to develop advice, having considered as much information from as many different sources as possible in the time available. It must arrive at a final position through wise judgements, balancing the many views it has heard, and it must lay out its reasoning in a transparent way, open to challenge by all.

THE NATURE AND CONTEXT OF PUBLIC INVOLVEMENT

 Public involvement in New Zealand has both negative and positive characteristics:

- worry about local services, which provokes attendance at meetings;
- anger or suspicion about the extent of health changes;
- interest and willingness to consider rationing issues;
- curiosity about the evidence for effective services;
- consultation cynicism and exhaustion;
- progressively more sophisticated engagement in the debate.

The rationing debate began as part of much wider health reforms, which resulted in significant changes to the existing structures for funding and provision of services. There has been, and still is, some suspicion about the government's overall intentions in its health and wider welfare changes. Since 1938, New Zealand has had a system of universal health service coverage on the basis of need, although not all services have been free. What was proposed in 1991 for health reforms was seen by many to be a major renegotiation of that social contract. Health professionals, health insurance providers and the media have a powerful role in informing public opinion. However, because of varying political and funding agendas and the restrictions of New Zealand's privacy legislation on full reporting of individual health stories, the discussion is often not fully informed or balanced.

Since 1992, public consultation on health questions has been extensive. Initially, a number of key agencies (the NHC, the Public Health Commission and the four regional health authorities) were all on the road at the same time, often consulting the same communities on what were seen to be very similar questions. The NHC, the Public Health Group of the Ministry of Health and the HFA are still running public consultations in 1998.

A large segment of the public has not been involved in any formal consultation activities. Given the time, the NHC budget and the staff available for consultation work, it would be an unaffordable ideal, even if people's own lack of interest did not make it impossible to achieve full public involvement. That does not mean people are not involved in the informal debate. A brief period of listening to talk-back radio on a health issue shows this!

It is difficult, therefore, to separate people's responses to specific rationing issues raised by the NHC from anxiety and suspicion about the purpose of the wider health reforms – and exhaustion at saying the same things many times to a large number of agencies. Much of the early feedback from communities raised issues that were outside the NHC's terms of reference.

NATIONAL HEALTH COMMITTEE FINDINGS

Community priorities

In 1992 the main focus of public involvement was on why rationing was necessary and what priorities communities had. *The Best of Health* (NHC 1992) was published and circulated widely. Broad comparisons or trade-offs were set out, identifying, for example, how many hip replacements or immunizations could be provided for the price of one heart transplant.

Six clear priorities emerged from general public consultation through town hall meetings and questionnaires. It was felt that more emphasis should be given to:

- mental health and substance abuse services;
- children's health services;
- integrated community care services, including culturally appropriate services responsive to Maori health needs;
- emergency ambulance services;
- hospice services;
- habilitation/rehabilitation services.

People wanted basic services available closer to home, shaped in ways which were more flexible and responsive to individual needs. Community rather than institutional care was preferred. Children, the elderly, and ethnic groups, particularly Maori, were important. Access to emergency services was important for people in rural areas. People felt there must be adequate support services for people disabled in accidents or after major illness, and for people who were dying. Disease prevention and health promotion were also important.

Communities were willing to make trade-offs. In particular, they emphasized quality of life rather than quantity of life, as a consistent theme. They supported a shift in resources towards improved basic care services before more extensive availability of high-tech services (MRI, CT scans, organ transplantation). They wanted to see more emphasis on community-located services in preference to in-patient care.

Of interest in 1998, those early priorities have translated into various policy and purchasing initiatives, which have given identified service areas increasing emphasis. Support has continued for their legitimacy. More latterly, as people's concerns are being addressed, other priorities are starting to emerge (such as a need for a focus on whole families, youth health, and adequate funding for people with disabilities). The challenge for policy makers and funders is to identify the next areas where worthwhile investments can be made while, at the same time, maintaining progress on the early priorities.

Philosophical framework for rationing decisions

In 1993, *The Best of Health 2* (NHC 1993a) asked the public how we should decide what services should be publicly funded. Substantial support emerged for the four-question framework for decision making about services, set out in that document:

- *benefit* or effectiveness of the services
  (does it do more good than harm?)
- *value for money* or cost-effectiveness
  (is the service sufficiently effective to justify the cost, especially if an equally effective but cheaper alternative is available?)
- *fairness* in access and use of the resource
  (is this the best way to use the resource or should it be used for a different service, or for someone else, or at some other time?)
- *consistency with communities' values*
  (are these the services most valued by communities?)[4]

The framework has been adopted by the committee and advised to the Minister of Health as the set of principles which should underpin all policy advice and health purchasing decisions, with the practical effect that resources should go to those who will receive the greatest likely benefit.

Definition of effective services

Public input into the rationing debate must be more than a view on general priorities or principles. In 1992–3, the committee undertook extensive work with clinicians, service providers and other experts, including public representatives, on specific treatments or service areas for both health and disability support, by way of consensus panels and contested public hearings. In the first two years, 18 topics were selected for detailed evaluation and consultation.[5]

Panels were asked to answer the following questions for each topic:

- How do we achieve the best health outcomes for users in this service area?
- How do we ensure that we are funding effective services which are the best use of scarce resources in this service area?
- What are priorities for resource allocation within this identified service area?

The consensus panels included a mixture of expert professional and community people, assisted by a facilitator. They provided independent advice to the committee on best practice, or guidelines for services under usual circumstances, on each of the topics.

This first wave of work has been added to significantly from 1994 through to the present. Service evaluations have occurred by means of contested hearings, often open to the public, expert advisory groups, and commissioned expert reports. All consensus conference or hearing reports have been subjected to peer review and wider public comment before adoption as committee advice to the Minister of Health.

In late 1995, the NHC was successful in persuading the government to fund an extended programme of work on best practice or service guidelines. The committee reasoned that an effective way to ensure rational, evidence-based practice was to make both providers and the public aware of the benefits, costs, harms and opportunity costs of treatment and that guidelines were a good way to help achieve this. From July 1996 to June 1999, the NHC's budget has been doubled to accelerate the progress on guidelines development and implementation.

Many community representatives have provided significant input to this detailed service evaluation work. For example, the advice on the use of hormone replacement therapy was agreed to by the consensus panel only after strenuous resistance from one of the consumer representatives who questioned whether a normal condition of life was being over-medicalized. Similarly, guidelines developed in areas such as mental health, blood pressure management and treatment for stomach ulcers (to name a few) have been thoroughly tested and are very practical and consumer friendly as a direct result of consumer (public) input.[6]

Focused public consultation through invited submissions

Findings from the early consensus conferences suggested that best outcomes would be achieved from some services in the following ways:

- When certain services were limited to *national or regional centres* (rather than local centres) – for example, kidney transplants, liver transplants, management of very low birthweight babies, heart bypass operations, angioplasty.
- By better *managing waiting times* through the development of agreed criteria for prioritizing patients according to their potential to benefit from services; establishing maximum appropriate waiting times; separating routine (elective) and acute medical and surgical cases into two streams, with routine cases given a 'booked' date for their operations. People not meeting the criteria would not be placed on waiting lists but would be referred back to their primary care practitioner for management.
- By developing *evidence-based practice guidelines* for treatments or services under usual circumstances which could increase consistency of practice, improve prescribing patterns and referral patterns, and promote clinical audit and continuing medical education – for example, hormone replacement therapy; management of raised blood pressure; management of dyspepsia.
- By encouraging a *holistic or integrated approach* to managing patient care as too often there is wasteful duplication of tests or diagnostic procedures, or people receive services, aids, or equipment unsuitable for different aspects of their lives (such as heavy wheelchairs which are easily used inside only).

These expert findings were taken to the wider public for consideration. A third public discussion document, *Seeking Consensus* (NHC 1993b), released widely in 1993, explored the implications of the approaches – people might have to travel away from home for some services, people who did not meet agreed criteria might be removed from current waiting lists, and primary care practitioners might have to follow explicit guidelines for some treatments under usual circumstances.

The committee received over 450 submissions from groups and individuals. Workshops were also held with groups of general practitioners around the country. Submissions were very largely in support of the four proposals. They formed the basis, therefore, of detailed service evaluation work in 1994, the subsequent extended guidelines programme (1996–9), and work in 1995–6 on priority criteria for access to elective surgical procedures and the development of booking systems (Hadorn and Holmes 1997).

Focus groups on ethical considerations in prioritizing health care

In the general public consultation activities undertaken by the committee in 1992–3, it was clear that the views of some groups in the community were not well represented. A focus group method was used in 1994 to consult people representing rural, urban low-income, older age, youth, Maori and Pacific Island interests and those of people with disabilities. The groups were asked about the meaning of 'fairness' and the ethical issues that emerge when health resource allocation decisions are made.[7]

All groups recognized the difficulties involved in such decisions. Two powerful shared values were concern for the vulnerable (the young or old) and the desire for co-operation, with all group members making whatever contribution they could. 'Need' emerged as the overwhelming consideration for the groups. It was accepted, however, that some should limit meeting their needs to ensure the welfare or survival of others. While much common ground was identified, it was also clear that different communities have some significant differences in their underlying values – something the NHC attempts to accommodate in its recommendations.

Public forums on the place of social factors in clinical priority criteria

In detailed work with professionals on determining priority for elective surgical procedures, it emerged that if there is only enough funding for operations for four people but five patients with similar clinical circumstances present, professionals use social factors (non-medical factors) to decide who should go first. Those factors may be used inconsistently and informally, however.

Panels of randomly selected members of the public, along with selected health professionals and managers were asked to debate:

- whether social factors should be considered;
- which ones are acceptable;
- how much weighting should be given to social factors compared with clinical judgement.

Specifically, the panels considered the place of social factors in decision making on access to coronary artery bypass grafting and angioplasty, and access to cataract surgery.[8] Conclusions from this initiative suggest that, for the public, a person's clinical condition, together with the likely outcome of any treatment, are the two most important aspects to consider when deciding who should get surgery. However, the panels agreed that social factors may have a place in deciding priorities.

In debating a set of scenarios of different people with different life circumstances, the health professionals present said they believed society accepts that a 38-year-old should get heart surgery ahead of an 83-year-old, all other things being equal. Panel members did not challenge this point. There was some support for the idea that people who did not take responsibility for their health – people who continued to smoke, who drank alcohol excessively, and who would not lose weight – should come second to those who did make an effort to stop or reduce those aspects of their behaviour. But others felt uncomfortable at imposing their values on other people. They believed that the influences on people's behaviour were complex and could not be reduced to notions of responsibility or irresponsibility.[9]

The committee concluded that the place and weighting of social factors in assessing priority is limited. Factors adopted following public consultation and still included in priority criteria in use in 1998 are *ability to work, give care to dependants or live independently*. They account for 10 per cent of the total priority score where they are used.

Advising on relative priorities between services

The process for developing the priority criteria themselves – that is the technical, clinical evaluation instruments – has not involved members of the public. However, the criteria can tell us clearly about levels of access and the cost of changing current access thresholds. That information *can* involve the public, and it can inform the debate on the relative priorities between services.

In the case of coronary artery bypass grafting (CABG), current access thresholds are set at 35 points, within existing levels of funding. Clinicians would prefer to be able to offer surgery at 25 points. Based on current numbers waiting and the cost of the operation, improved access to a threshold of 25 points would involve an additional $6 million per year for this service alone. Some of the additional cost would be offset by reduced doctor visits and drugs but, arguably, greater clarity about access levels might also increase rates of referral for CABG procedures. Descriptions of the degree of pain or functional disability people face at different access levels have been prepared so members of the public can understand what the health condition of heart patients might be like.[10] They can then debate whether the conditions and likely benefit are sufficient to justify moving $6m from other services to improve access to CABG.

In public consultations in 1997 and 1998, the NHC has been able to use this example, and others, to begin debating with the public the appropriateness of the current balance and mix of existing services, and where changes might be made in the relative priority of services to achieve better health outcomes. Although it is still early days, it is clear when talking to people with disabilities or mental health problems, or families with medically fragile or chronically ill children, for example, that the case for improved access to CABG comes a poor second to other priorities.

Ongoing processes to be used for prioritizing services

From 1994–6, NHC work focused heavily on technical service evaluations. There has been little opportunity truly to engage the wider public – despite the presence of consumer representatives on service effectiveness panels and the call for public submissions. 1997–8 has seen the beginning of two significant initiatives to increase the involvement of the public in detailed rationing discussions.

First, *The Best of Health 3* was published in late 1997 (NHC 1997) to take the public debate onto the next level – beyond 'Why do we need to ration?' and 'What principles should we use?' to 'What processes should be used to prioritize publicly funded services?' *The*

Best of Health 3, coalescing six years of committee work, makes four points:

- rationing of health services is inevitable;
- the processes for making rationing decisions must be transparent;
- communities must be involved – their values are essential when rationing decisions mean that not everyone will get all the health services they want;
- there are transparent tools – guidelines and priority criteria – which can help the decisions.

Public comment is invited on the value of transparent processes and tools. Should rationing decisions be open? How might we achieve more explicit, open and transparent processes – which necessarily imply the greater involvement of the public along with professionals – to inform rationing discussions? Do people agree that guidelines or priority criteria are a way to decide what services should be publicly funded, and for whom? The public is also challenged to think about the evidence for effectiveness of services, the balance between prevention/promotion, personal health treatments or disability support services, whether we should strive for cure at all costs compared with care – and it asks for public views on whether we should always try to defy death. Consultations are still proceeding and early indications are for support of the committee's four points.

In the second initiative, a public dimension is to be added to the substantial programme of work the NHC has initiated with health and disability professionals in guidelines development. Consumer training programmes are to be run to increase the numbers of public participants in guidelines development work and to help establish a network of citizens interested and skilled in consumer representation as part of guidelines panels. The aim is to enhance consumers' skills in putting forward their perspective on health services – after all, they are the ones who live with the outcomes of those services.

There is a significant level of enthusiasm for this initiative which is seen as ground-breaking with respect to consumer representation within the health sector in New Zealand and more generally. The committee expects to run a number of consumer training courses in 1998–9. Public representatives would then be linked into guidelines development activity increasingly occurring out in the sector, spearheaded by professionals themselves, with only a watching brief from the NHC.

CONCLUSION

This is a progress report on involving the public in health care rationing. Much of the NHC's work has been qualitative rather than quantitative. Very few NHC initiatives have involved carefully designed research studies in the strictest sense, with 'before' and 'after' evaluations. In NHC's view, that does not mean the lessons are any less important for a wider understanding of how to make hard choices.

Rationing or prioritizing of health care is definitely on the public agenda in New Zealand. The debate is highlighted when there is media coverage of the impact of rationing decisions on individuals. The news coverage of decisions to decline renal dialysis to two men – whose situations were extensively debated in the media – was a lightning rod for public opinion about health rationing. Even for people who accept, in principle, the need to make such decisions, when an identifiable individual is denied a service in accordance with those decisions it is very hard not to be moved.

Public demand is growing for the government to increase expenditure in health, even at the expense of proposed tax cuts. But there is no easy answer to what is the correct amount to spend on health services. It is inescapable that even if total spending on health were to double, public funding always runs out at some point. Decisions still need to be made on the margins of funding. Despite funding increases, pressures will still continue as health care improvements outpace economic growth.

Public confidence that 'health services will be there for people when they need them' may be undermined when the realities of hard choices are made public. Is that a reason to muddle through and not be explicit? The NHC thinks not. It has been promoting public and professional participation in rationing of health care for almost seven years. Understanding and ownership of the need to make such decisions is vital both among health providers and members of the public. It must be a shared and open debate with all the interested parties.

The role of the media is vital in having a better informed public discussion on the issues. In some cases, I believe that the New Zealand public has been badly served by the media. Health stories often focus on the exceptions. Sensational headlines frequently do not reflect the content of the stories. Significantly also, the media are constrained by privacy laws from being able to report fully.

Are we having the broad, informed, rational debate that is

needed? The honest answer is no, not yet. But the NHC believes that there is greater recognition of the issues and acceptance of the need to make rationing choices, particularly among some health professionals and the more thoughtful media commentators who have a strong influence on public opinion.

There are no single or simple answers to this dilemma which hold for all time. A list of 'core' services is too static – with the rate of technological progress, lists are out of date before the ink is dry! Simply listing services also implies a guarantee of access. It does not allow account to be taken of individual circumstances and the relative degree of benefit people might obtain. Communities' priorities also change over time. They need continual review and renegotiation as evidence emerges for new procedures or as evidence changes about the benefits or harms of existing services.

Rationing requires the constant juggling of many priorities. The rationing process must balance wants, needs, rights, ability to benefit, possible harms, and competing claims on all the resources available for health care. Regardless of the level at which decisions are made within the health sector, every single decision involves a trade-off for another service or another person at another time. There are about 60,000 people working in the New Zealand health sector. There are 3.8 million potential service users. Clearly it is impossible to direct every decision to be made. Provided the decisions aim to achieve the most cost-effective and fair outcomes for the part of the sector involved, the totality of decisions should add up to a well-functioning sector which is sophisticated and responsive.

Public engagement is important in customizing services to local circumstances – and to achieve understanding of the trade-offs or compromises which may be necessary. On more technical matters, it is important to cut a course between expecting people to make decisions about matters that are extremely complex, requiring an understanding of a great deal of specialized information, and leaving the community out in the cold. That is a delicate path to pick. But the counterweight to having the authority and responsibility to give advice affecting others is the requirement to be accountable for that advice, and to arrive at the advice in a way that is explicit, honest, transparent – where the reasoning or workings can be shown – so that the public can know that the best option has been taken in the light of available evidence or information.

Finally, if I may focus on the NHC's most recent practical initiative in involving the public, the committee's consumer training programme in guidelines development should raise public engagement by several notches. As a case study, warts and all in these early days, it shows some promise. New Zealand is a small country with a small population. People share their experiences. They talk with their families, friends and communities. They are increasingly informed about health matters, via the media and the Internet. Their views may be well informed or their expectations and hopes may be raised falsely or unrealistically. And they certainly let their views be known in various ways.

The National Health Committee believes – and is striving to put into practice – that we should value the interest of the New Zealand public. They rightly want to know what services will be publicly funded for them, who makes those decisions and how they are made. It is important to harness that public energy to achieve effective, fair and understandable decision making about rationing of health care.

NOTES

1 The National Health Committee (full title: National Advisory Committee on Health and Disability) was originally established in March 1992 as the National Advisory Committee on Core Health and Disability Support Services, known as the Core Services Committee. In 1996, the brief of the committee was expanded to cover advice on priorities for public health services, in addition to advice on personal health services and disability support services. The committee's name changed at that time.

2 Some public commentators argue that trade-offs or reductions in services can be avoided if additional funding is made available. They give no view on the health funding level they prefer, its affordability or its priority in relation to other areas of social spending. As New Zealand's economy has improved since 1992, significant injections of new money have been allocated for health services. The government remains concerned, however, about the long-term sustainability of the funding path for health. Thus, the focus for NHC work remains: that health resources are ultimately always finite and rationing choices will need to be made on the margins of health funding, even though periodically there may be some increase in overall levels.

3 The initiative for establishing the committee to lead the rationing debate in New Zealand came from a National (conservative) government with a strong agenda to achieve greater clarity about what health care the state would be responsible for and what individuals would need to take care of for themselves. There is no cross-party consensus on this issue. Although the main opposition party (Labour) acknowledges that there are finite health resources and choices will be made on

how to use them, it is less clear about its position on an explicit public debate on health rationing. Other parties deny that rationing is necessary, preferring to solve the issue of growing demand by proposing to raise taxes. There is no acknowledgement in this position that choices would still have to be made, even on the margins of additional funding from higher taxes.

4 In translation from policy advice to government requirements of the sector, the principles have been expressed using different although congruent terms – effectiveness, efficiency, equity, acceptability.

5 Topics were chosen to cover a range of significant health areas. The treatments involved high total costs; there was public concern about the issue; there was adequate information available; and there was a good chance of reaching consensus on issues which would make a difference. Many of the topics derived from an analysis of the 20 most common kinds of hospital discharge diagnosis and the 20 kinds of hospital discharge diagnosis that cost the most in total. The 18 topics are major joint replacement (hip and knee); coronary artery bypass graft surgery and angioplasty; management of end-stage kidney failure; management of the baby under 1000 grams; management of raised blood pressure; aftercare of normal delivery; prescribing minor tranquillizers; management of major psychoses; early detection of breast cancer; well-child care; disability support services – priorities; self-assessment – a process for older people; self-help and empowerment for people with disabilities; client orientation of services; living at home; hormone replacement therapy; management of dyspepsia; and treatment for drug and alcohol problems.

6 The committee's expanded work programme in guidelines development and implementation and its service evaluation reviews from 1994 to 1998 have resulted in publications on the following topics. *Delivery of Health Services to Smaller Communities*; *Costs and Effectiveness of Infertility Services: A Decision Analysis; Priorities for Genetic Services*; *Care for Older People*; He Anga Whakamana: *A Framework for the Delivery of Disability Support Services for Maori*; *Habilitation and Rehabilitation*; *Guidelines for the Treatment and Management of Depression by Primary Health Care Professionals* (including a summary for professionals and consumer pamphlets); consumer pamphlets on peptic ulcers; *Prostate Cancer Screening* (professional and consumer guides); *Acute Low Back Pain Guide* and *Guide to Assessing Psychosocial Yellow Flags in Acute Low Back Pain* (plus consumer pamphlet); *The Prevention, Recognition and Management of Young People at Risk of Suicide: A Guide for Schools*; *Prevention of Falls in Older Populations – in the Community, and in Institutional Settings*; *Preventive Dental Strategies for Older Populations*; *Prevention of Osteoporosis* (plus consumer pamphlet); *Who Is Responsible for the Provision of Support Services for People with Disabilities?*; *Guidelines for the Surgical Management of Breast Cancer*; *Primary Prevention of Cardiovascular Disease in Older New Zealanders*; *Memory Loss: Is it Alzheimer's or a Related Dementia?*

7 Groups debated the meaning of 'fairness' in setting priorities, using three scenarios:
   - dividing up a birthday cake;
   - sharing food supplies under a war-time state of siege with a group of people of different gender, age, mental and physical ability, with one woman breastfeeding a baby; and
   - survival of that same group of people in a lifeboat which would take ten days to row to shore, with food for only four days.

   The implications for setting health priorities were then discussed.

8 Social factors included the following: young family; working for wages; will not lose weight; unemployed; sole income earner for family; single; pain and discomfort comes on with activity or stress; no family to help out; job is threatened; has health insurance; has already had coronary bypass surgery (and would benefit from it again); doesn't have long to live because of other health problems; continues to smoke; care giving (looking after a frail parent or dependent children); can't enjoy leisure activity (playing with grandchildren, tramping, fishing, walking, playing bowls); age. The factors were a mixture of negative and positive characteristics, and some factors may be argued to be a justifiable clinical consideration (for example, age, as a proxy for general physical condition, or the presence of other diseases or disabilities, which may compromise the effectiveness of some interventions).

9 There is ongoing debate about the inclusion of age/life expectancy, and health status/other significant disease as valid clinical considerations. This may be resolved late in 1998. Clinical judgements about the most effective use of resources must take account of the frailty of age or co-morbidity in assessing likely outcomes for some procedures. Many believe it is a waste of scarce resources if a person stands to gain no or very little clinical benefit from a procedure. However, discrimination on the basis of age or pre-existing health conditions may be in contravention of current Human Rights legislation in New Zealand. An amendment is planned for the Human Rights Act 1993 to clarify that sound rationing (different treatment) is lawful where it is based on an assessment of need or ability to benefit and has regard to the best health that is reasonably achievable within the amount of health funding available.

10 **Typical patient profiles**
   55 points or more – markedly reduced quality of life, chest pain and breathlessness with almost any physical activity. Reduction of life expectancy of one to two years without surgery.
   35–54 points – much reduced quality of life. Pain on exertion (e.g. walking one to two blocks). Moderately reduced life expectancy of eight to twelve months without surgery.
   25–34 points – intermittent pain and breathlessness when walking or climbing stairs rapidly. Modest reduction in life expectancy of four to eight months without surgery.

17

EXPLICIT RATIONING, DEPRIVATION DISUTILITY AND DENIAL DISUTILITY: EVIDENCE FROM A QUALITATIVE STUDY

Joanna Coast

DEPRIVATION DISUTILITY AND DENIAL DISUTILITY

There are many important issues to debate concerning the process of health care rationing, one of which is the question of whether rationing should be implicit or explicit (Coast 1997; Doyal 1997). Implicit rationing can be defined as the limitation of care in which neither the decisions about which forms of care are provided nor the bases for those decisions are clearly expressed: it is the un-acknowledged limitation of care. Explicit rationing is the opposite, with clarity in both the decisions made about the provision of care and the reasons for those decisions (Coast *et al.* 1996). A system in which rationing was wholly implicit would be at one end of a con-tinuum, at the other end of which would be a system in which rationing was wholly explicit. These rationing decisions may be made at different levels ranging from decisions across entire ser-vices to decisions at the level of the individual patient. In practice, both implicit and explicit decisions are made. Rationing in the UK has traditionally been implicit (Aaron and Schwarz 1984; Grimes 1987), although there is increasingly both pressure to change (New 1996) and actual explicitness in some decision making (Redmayne *et al.* 1993).

Reasons have been advanced both for and against explicitness in health care rationing. Commentators have argued for explicitness on the grounds of both an ideological belief in openness, honesty and democracy (Doyal 1997) and a perception that explicit rationing will allow particular principles to be followed, ensuring that the scarce resources available for health care are used in the best ways possible (an idea particularly linked with the economist's notion of maximizing health gain) (New 1996). In contrast, arguments have been advanced against explicit rationing on the grounds that it is not possible to obtain consensus about principles (Klein 1993a), that it is not possible to sustain explicit rationing because it will cause instability within the health care system (Hunter 1993; Mechanic 1995), and that there is the potential for increased disutility for citizens caused by feelings of deprivation and denial (Coast 1997). This chapter concentrates on the latter issue.

Previous work by this author has suggested that implementing explicit rationing policies may potentially have some disbenefit or, to use the economists' terminology, disutility, which has not commonly been considered (Coast 1997). Such disutility could arise in one of two ways. First, there is the potential for individuals, as citizens, to experience disutility as a result of being asked to partake in the process of denying treatment or care to other members of society. Second, there is the potential for individuals, as patients, to experience disutility as a result of being told explicitly that their own health treatment or care is being rationed.

Why might these forms of disutility arise? In the first case, of denial disutility, it is believable that explicitly denying treatment to patients who are sick and who may die or live with severe disability could be expected to cause the individuals making that decision considerable disutility. Indeed, Aaron and Schwartz have shown that doctors themselves avoid making these decisions explicit by gradually and implicitly adjusting their perception of medical need to coincide with available resources (Aaron and Schwarz 1984). In the second case, of deprivation disutility, it is suggested that disutility arises from knowing that something could have been done but was not. This is a notion developed by two economists in relation to feelings of deprivation resulting from a failure to receive antenatal screening followed by the birth of a baby with a condition that could have been detected with such screening (Mooney and Lange 1993). The analogous rationing situation is that individuals might feel grievance if they know that a treatment exists but that they themselves are unable to access it for financial reasons. They may also feel resentment towards those who do receive treatment as well as losing hope for their own situation.

The important question in relation to these forms of disutility is whether such disutility could outweigh any potential advantages (increases in utility) associated with a move from implicit to explicit rationing. The aim of this research was therefore to explore whether there is any empirical basis for these two theoretical concepts among citizens.

METHODS

This study was conducted within the wider context of an exploration of the citizen's utility function as it relates to both health care and health care rationing. The use of qualitative methods was considered appropriate for three main reasons. First, the issues to be discussed were complex and concerned with meaning, hence unlikely to be captured through simple survey questions. Second, preferences concerning health care rationing are unlikely to be fully formed among many citizens, who may have had little contact with health care services and may therefore require time for reflection and discussion. Third, in the formation of survey questions, a decision (value judgement) must be made about the content of those questions, yet this implies a potential imposition of the views of the economist on the content of the utility function, which would be considered inappropriate by at least some economists (Evans and Wolfson 1980).

Initial fieldwork was undertaken in the form of focus groups with members of the public sampled both from interest groups and randomly from the electoral roll. Informants were located in one UK county and comprised individuals living in a city and in a small town. The primary aim of the focus groups was to discuss whether the public should be involved in health care decision making. From these focus groups participants were purposively selected for interview based on their comments in the group and with the intention of obtaining a broad range of views about the extent to which individuals appeared to want to participate in health care decision making. Semi-structured interviews were then conducted with 14 informants. Interviews lasted between 30 minutes and one hour. Topics were discussed as they arose during the interview and covered the following issues: important aspects of health care; who should make choices in health care and why; whether the informant would want to participate in health care decision making; whether the informant perceived health care as being rationed; and whether the informant would want to know about any rationing of their own care.

All interviews were tape recorded, fully transcribed and each transcript checked for accuracy; tape failure for one interview meant that the findings were based on data from 13 informants. Analysis drew on grounded theory procedures (Strauss and Corbin 1990). Fieldnotes were made following each interview, with memos written as appropriate. Categories and sub-categories were developed, modified and extended on the basis of emerging themes as the analysis was conducted. The technique of 'questioning' (Strauss and Corbin 1990) was used to enhance theoretical sensitivity while developing categories and sub-categories, and the aim was to accommodate all meaningful phrases. Detailed descriptive accounts were formed for each individual, and matrices were then used to facilitate comparison and contrast between individuals. Five major themes were then described across all citizen informants with the aim of providing a full explanation taking into account negative cases.

FINDINGS

This chapter presents findings focusing on the specific issues relating to deprivation and denial disutility as defined above. These findings are drawn from two categories developed during the analysis: 'choosing' and 'knowing'. The findings are illustrated with verbatim quotes from the informants. The findings do not seek to be statistically representative of citizens and cannot be generalized quantitatively. Instead they are intended to illuminate and explore the issues surrounding deprivation disutility and denial disutility.

Denial disutility/'choosing'

There was wide variation among the citizen informants in the extent to which they wanted to partake in making rationing choices in health care. It appeared from the discussions with these informants that they could be conceptualized as falling into three groups (of similar size) relating to the extent to which they wanted to participate in these decisions. At one extreme, there was a group of individuals who were unequivocal in their view that they were strongly opposed to having any personal involvement in such decisions. At the other extreme was a group of individuals who were unequivocal in their willingness to be involved in health care decision making even if this would mean the denial of care to particular individuals. In the middle was a group of informants who were more equivocal in their views about whether they wanted to be involved in health care decision making, but who showed considerable reluctance to make decisions that would result in the denial of treatment to individuals. Findings relating to these specific groups are detailed below.

Unequivocally opposed to involvement in health care rationing

Informants in this group were extremely reluctant to take part in health care rationing. Decisions were likened to sending someone to the gallows or playing Russian roulette, and some informants became extremely agitated at the thought of having to make these decisions:

> No, I just wouldn't, no I don't know why, I just, how would you decide? I wouldn't know how to decide . . . I wouldn't be able to decide which things should get the money, no, and I wouldn't want to, you know I wouldn't.
>
> (Female informant, aged 50)

The extreme reluctance of these informants to take any part whatsoever in health care decision making seems to relate to three main areas. First, they perceived the decisions to be extremely complex, such that a large degree of medical expertise is required:

> I mean it would need a doctor to say, you know, if this money . . . was put in here these people could be cured.
>
> (Female informant, aged 50)

> . . . what society might decide, might *not* necessarily be the best thing because they are not *involved* . . . the doctors, or the specialists, they would be the best ones to make the decision . . . because they are professionals.
>
> (Male informant, aged 31)

Second, they perceived the decisions to be extremely difficult, in the sense that they would have to weigh the competing claims for treatment by different individuals. They found it difficult to formulate mechanisms for deciding between such competing claims:

I'm saying that cosmetic surgery is a big issue, if it affects self esteem yes, but . . . you can say . . . a 70-year-old person would . . . want to look like a 30-year-old person, because of their self esteem, so it's very hard . . .

(Male informant, aged 48)

And how do you decide? I knew that was . . . that's it, so how do you decide? . . . Oh dear. Here we are back again with the the crunch question aren't we?

(Female informant, aged 50)

Third, they appeared to feel unable to cope with any responsibility for the decisions that are made, suggesting that such decisions would weigh heavily upon their conscience:

. . . because maybe I can't cope with it. I mean I think there are some situations in life that you feel you don't want to know about, well certainly I've learned this, perhaps it's self-protection in a way.

(Female informant, aged 68)

Equivocal about involvement in health care rationing

In many ways those who were equivocal about involvement in health care rationing were similar to those informants who did not want to participate in such decision making. They appeared to be almost as reluctant to be involved, but a small part of them seemed to have some interest in being, or desire to be, involved. In general they exhibited greater conflict between wanting to participate and not wanting to participate:

So, perhaps I would be a little bit put off by having to make such a decision, I wouldn't mind listening in though.

(Male informant, aged 71)

. . . I'd like to put my views . . . but I don't know if I could be the one saying yea or nay.

(Female informant, aged 33)

The reasons for not wanting involvement in health care decision making were also very similar: a perception of insufficient expertise; a tendency to view the decisions as difficult (although to a lesser extent than among those unequivocal about not wanting to participate); and a desire to protect oneself from the decision. The greatest difference between the two groups was in the views expressed on expertise. Although this group expressed doubts that they, as members of the public, had sufficient expertise to make decisions, there was not as a result the automatic acceptance of the medical profession as the appropriate decision makers. There appeared to be internal conflict within this group between a personal desire to avoid responsibility and a perception that decisions should not perhaps be left entirely to the medical profession.

Unequivocally willing to be involved in health care rationing

Members of this group were quite unequivocal in their desire to be involved in decision making, with some suggestion that they would be willing to go as far as taking reponsibility for the decisions that were made:

> I mean it's like jury service isn't it? I've done that and I enjoyed doing it and it seems to be the right way of doing things . . . if . . . you chose twelve people, put them in a room and two groups of society were presenting you with two aspects of someone's case or two priorities and we were having to make a choice between the two, yes, I would be willing to do it on that basis.
>
> (Male informant, aged 63)

Members of this group showed very different characteristics from those in the other groups. Among these informants expertise was perceived as resulting from life experiences, with medical expertise being viewed as both less important and more attainable than by members of the other two groups. None of the informants in this group perceived the decisions that have to be made as particularly difficult, and they showed a tendency to trust in their own judgements:

> When I say well look we've made this decision . . . because of these facts and if it's clear cut like that then it's easy isn't it, it's not pleasant, but it's easy.
>
> (Male informant, aged 65)

Deprivation disutility/'knowing'

In contrast to the findings above, there was considerably less variation in views among informants about whether they wanted to know about any rationing of their own health care. Although there was a small amount of ambiguity (wanting to know about some decisions but not others) among two informants, almost all informants showed a strong preference for knowing if their own care was being rationed:

> I mean they can come out with all this sort of thing when at the bottom line it is all about money. Now I would much sooner be told.
>
> (Female informant, aged 62)

There was, however, the suggestion from some informants that others may not want to know about the rationing of care, with informants likening the information to that of a terminal prognosis where there appears to be variation in what individuals want to know. Most informants suggested reasons for wanting to know about the rationing of their own care. These reasons included wanting a good explanation for the decision (potentially linked with an appraisal by themselves as to whether the decision was correct or not), being able to protest against the decision and not wanting to give such power to doctors:

> ... if there is a decision made I'd like to maybe have some understanding *why* that decision was made, in terms of the technical side of it, you know, it might be just on a *tech*nical basis – you know there's no hope, 'You can have this expensive drug, but I can assure you it's not going to make any difference' ... and the *risks* involved, and then so maybe I could weigh it up and decide whether they were right.
>
> (Male informant, aged 31)

> Well if I know about it perhaps I could kick up a fuss and get it. If I don't know, then there's no chance at all, if you do know there might be some chance.
>
> (Male informant, aged 65)

Informants also spoke about how they might react to the knowledge that their care was being rationed. Here there was some difference of opinion, with some informants suggesting that they would accept the decision and others suggesting that they would make efforts to obtain treatment either through protest or through payment. Two informants had each experienced knowing about the rationing of their own care. In one case the individual had protested (unsuccessfully) and in the other the individual had paid for treatment:

> Because we're all selfish when it comes to that one. When it's you and your family, that's really all you're interested in, at that moment ... we *are* selfish because you read and hear of cases where you disagree with what they're doing.
>
> (Male informant, aged 65)

Implicit in these data is the view for many individuals that, at the point where their own care is being rationed, they cease to take a 'citizen' or societal view, and instead take a 'patient' or individual view of the situation.

DISCUSSION

These findings provide some support for the existence of denial disutility and deprivation disutility, with apparently stronger evidence for the existence of denial disutility. There is wide variation between the views of individuals, but at least one, and possibly two, groups of citizens seem likely to experience some element of denial disutility if they are asked to take responsibility for the rationing of health care. The views of individuals about whether they want to know about the rationing of health care provide some insight into the potential for deprivation disutility. The almost unanimous desire of individuals to know about any rationing of their own care suggests that deprivation disutility is not likely to be of great importance in the discussion about whether rationing should be implicit or explicit.

ACKNOWLEDGEMENTS

I would like to thank the following: Jenny Donovan and Stephen Frankel for helpful comments on this chapter; participants at the Second International Conference on Priority Setting in Health Care for comments on the presentation that preceded this chapter; and the following individuals who have been involved in the larger project, funded by South and West NHS Research and Development Directorate, from which informants were drawn for this particular research: Andrea Litva, Jenny Donovan, Jo Tacchi, Kieran Morgan, Mike Shepherd, John Eyles, Julia Abelson, Will Warin, Charlotte Baxter.

PART VII

RATIONING SPECIFIC TREATMENTS

18

PRIORITY SETTING IN PRACTICE

Sian Griffiths, John Reynolds and Tony Hope

This chapter provides a case study for priority setting in practice within an English health authority. It describes the process which has been developed, the ethical framework which underpins the decision-making process and the application in practice with specific reference to new and expensive drugs.

BACKGROUND

Oxfordshire Health Authority is responsible for the health of the population of the 600,000 people who live in the county. The county is predominantly rural, with a population dispersed between market towns and the countryside. There are two urban conurbations – Banbury in the north of the country and Oxford city. The relative affluence of the county coupled with the high standards and wide range of the services provided by the university hospitals are reflected in the health statistics which show a healthier than average population. However, the funding base has, for some years, been under the target allocation which the district could have expected to receive from the application of the national funding formula. This, as well as the opportunities of a system often working at the leading edge of medical science and the articulate nature of the population, have made it a necessity to be increasingly clear about the choices between treatments which have to be made. Priority setting – or rationing – has become explicit over recent years.

Although initially we were expected to devise a rational system based on analysis of relative merits of various treatments, like others (Holm 1998), we have increasingly recognized the complexity of the process, the poverty of comparable data and hence the need to focus on the process of priority setting itself.

The process which we have developed in the county focuses on the Priorities Forum. The forum is a sub-committee of the health authority and reports its decisions to their public meetings. With a membership across sectors and disciplines it is a representative body for the various interests across the county, including the public. It considers a wide range of issues: the introduction of new drugs, innovative treatments and individual exceptional needs. The outcomes of its deliberations are distributed widely to interested parties across the county, particularly to primary care. The initial stimulus for the creation of the Priorities Forum lay in the market reforms of the early 1990s and the introduction of contracts. This was accompanied by a parallel introduction of extra-contractual referrals for treatments not covered by the contracts. As a tertiary centre, Oxford could have expected to be the recipient of contractual flows from other counties.

However, there were certain groups of patients who needed to be referred out of the county for care, most notably those with mental health needs. The health authority board became anxious about the level of expenditure on these patients and the Priorities Forum began to meet to scrutinize these cases.

It became apparent that the decisions being made were often inconsistent, and this made it difficult to defend the choices being made. This led to the development of the ethical framework, which we describe later.

Using the ethical framework as a guide, individual cases were appraised in a consistent way which allowed us to derive a kind of 'case law'. The impact of this meant that many extra contractual referral (ECR) decisions could be made without reference to the forum, who increasingly began to consider some of the issues within specialties and, where possible, between clinical specialties and other areas of care.

Involvement of clinicians is key to the way that the forum works. Experience has taught us that preparation for discussion is essential if we are to avoid emotional shroud waving. For this reason, prior to attendance, clinicians are briefed that discussions will take place against the notion of an envelope of resource and the ethical framework.

ENVELOPE OF RESOURCE

With the rapid advance of technology, clinicians are often keen to introduce new treatments. Decisions about new areas of treatment are made within the framework of existing clinical practice – the envelope of resource.

Clinicians are asked to consider three questions:

1 If you want something outside your current fixed envelope of resource, can it be done by substituting a treatment of less value?
2 If demand for your service is increasing, what criteria are you using to agree the threshold of treatment?
3 If you do not believe that it is possible either to draw thresholds of care or to substitute treatment then which service might you give a smaller resource to in order for you to enlarge yours?

These are not easy questions and the debate is often less structured than this approach may imply, but it is used consistently so forum members can attempt to be fair. The approach has led to substitution of some treatments – for example, the dermatologists decided to introduce treatment of acne with isoretinoin and stop treating hirsutism. There are many examples of thresholds being drawn. Examples range from increasing the threshold for symptoms which would result in a coronary artery bypass to explicit recognition that children exhibiting general behavioural problems in school could no longer be seen by child and adolescent psychiatrists. This was a direct result of the impact of cuts in the social care budget.

The purpose of the third question is to raise the awareness of the complexity of the task of the health authority – making sure limited resources provide maximum health gain to the total population of the county in the most open, explicit and fair way possible. It has helped clinicians to see the issue as one of distributing money between services rather than as a battle between a clinical service and a mean health authority.

ETHICS FRAMEWORK

As the Priorities Forum developed it became increasingly clear that an ethical framework was needed, the three main reasons being:

1 To help in structuring discussion and to ensure that the important points were properly considered.
2 To ensure consistency of decision making, both from one meeting to another and with respect to decisions concerning different clinical settings.
3 To enable the forum to articulate the reasons for its decisions. This is particularly important for a proper appeals procedure and in the event of a decision coming under legal scrutiny. In such circumstances the courts are likely to consider whether the process and the grounds for making the decision were reasonable. An ethics framework is particularly important in judging the reasonableness of the grounds on which the decision was made.

The Forum set up an ethics sub-group which developed the first draft of the framework in the light both of the principal theories underlying resource allocation, and the forum's previous decisions. The draft framework was the subject of a day workshop for members of the forum and other senior members of the health authority. The framework was revised in the light of the feedback and experience of this workshop.

The ethics framework is structured around three main components.

Evidence of effectiveness

The framework distinguishes four aspects:

1 *Effectiveness* – the extent to which a treatment (or other health care intervention) achieves a desired effect (for example, the proportion of patients who would be expected to show the effect).
2 *Value* – a judgement as to the value of that effect in the relevant individual patient relative to the value of other treatments. A treatment which saves the life of young adults and restores them to full fitness is of high value. A treatment that removes a slight blemish from an unexposed part of the body would normally be of low value. More is said about this under equity below.
3 *Impact* – the value of an intervention weighted for the degree of effectiveness.
4 *Efficiency* – the impact per unit cost.

The purpose of these definitions is to clarify the distinction between value judgements and factual statements.

In deciding the priority of a health care intervention the framework considers that the evidence of effectiveness is of major importance. This evidence can fall broadly within three categories:

1 There is good evidence that the treatment is not effective.
2 There is good evidence that the treatment is effective.
3 The evidence either way is not good.

Clearly treatment which falls into the first category should not be funded. Treatments that fall into the second category may or may not be funded depending on efficiency (as defined above). Many treatments (or other health care interventions) fall into the third category. In such cases many clinicians may believe that the treatment is valuable but large, well-designed trials have not been carried out. It could be said for treatments in this third category that there is no good evidence for effectiveness. However, they should not be confused with the first category. It is desirable to obtain good quality evidence about effectiveness, and research aimed at obtaining such evidence should be encouraged. However, when evidence is poor then the forum has to make a judgement about the likely effectiveness in the knowledge that good quality evidence is not available.

In judging the quality of evidence the priorities forum will often need the advice of those expert in the area, such as senior clinicians. When seeking advice the forum requires, from the adviser, a full declaration of interests relevant to the advice given.

Equity

The basic principle of equity is that people in similar situations should be treated similarly. For this reason it is important that there is consistency in the way in which decisions are reached at different times and in different settings.

This principle of equity also requires that there is no discrimination on grounds irrelevant to priority for health care. The ethical framework identifies a number of grounds that do not justify difference in priority: race, social position, financial status, religion or place of abode (within the area covered by the health authority). It also states that there should be no discrimination on the following grounds: age, employment status, family circumstances, lifestyle and learning disability. However, this statement needs some qualification. The features in the second list may affect aspects of the health care intervention which should (in the view of the forum) affect priority. For example, an older person may have less to gain from an intervention because of a likely shorter time to benefit; a self-employed person may have more to lose by waiting for treatment than a retired person. While it might be legitimate for an individual clinician to ensure that a particular self-employed person was treated more quickly for a non-urgent treatment than a retired person, it would very rarely be right for the health authority to make such a judgement. This is because such a judgement requires a great deal of knowledge about the circumstances of both people – knowledge that would rarely be available to the health authority.

In developing the principles on which equity is based the forum considered in particular two broad approaches. One approach is that of maximizing the welfare of patients within the budget available. The second is giving priority to those in most need. Neither approach by itself was considered adequate. The maximization of welfare takes no direct account of how that welfare is distributed between different people. Equity would seem to require giving some priority to those in most need even if this does not produce the greatest level of welfare overall. The forum tries to balance these approaches using a two-step process. First it considers cost-effectiveness of the intervention under consideration e.g. on the basis of QALYs. Second, if the intervention is less cost-effective than those normally funded, it considers whether there are, nevertheless, reasons for funding it. Relevant reasons include:

- urgent need (e.g. immediately life-saving treatment);
- treatment for those whose quality of life is severely affected by chronic illness (e.g. due to a severely incapacitating neurological condition);
- whether the high expense of the treatment is due to characteristics of the patient that should not affect priority. One example is that the same level of dental care should be available to people with learning disabilities as with the normal population, even if it is less cost-effective because more specialized services are needed.

Patient choice

Respecting patients' wishes and enabling patients to have control over their health care are considered by the forum to be important values. The value of patient choice has three implications for the work of the forum.

1 In assessing research on the effectiveness of a treatment it is important that the outcome measures used in the research include those which matter to patients.
2 Within those health care interventions that are purchased, patients should be enabled to make their own choices about which they want.
3 Each patient is unique. Good quality evidence about the effectiveness of an intervention normally addresses outcomes in a large group of people. There may be a good reason to believe that a particular patient stands to gain significantly more from the intervention than most of those who formed the study group in the relevant research. This may justify a particular patient receiving treatment not normally provided.

However, the authority will not make an exception to a decision not to purchase a particular intervention simply because a patient wishes to have that intervention. This is on the grounds of equity: one patient's choice is another patient's lack of choice.

THE APPLICATION OF THE ETHICS FRAMEWORK: NEW DRUGS

When a new drug is licensed the manufacturers have to provide extensive evidence to demonstrate safety, efficacy and a quality of production. Even so, at the time of launch, the safety data are always incomplete, and there is little or no real-life experience in general patient populations not represented in carefully supervised clinical trials. Recent experience with several new drugs which have been withdrawn from use on safety grounds demonstrates the need for caution on behalf of purchasers and prescribers.

Thirty or more new drugs are licensed and launched in the UK every year and the Priorities Forum is frequently approached by Trusts and clinicians with requests for increased funding to permit the introduction of new drugs. The process whereby evaluation is undertaken may vary depending on the clinical context, but the ethics framework is always central to the ultimate decision. The process undertaken in Oxford for riluzole (a drug used for the treatment of motor neurone disease) and isotretinoin (a vitamin A derivative used in the treatment of severe acne) has been described previously (Hope *et al.* 1998). When donepezil (Aricept (r), an inhibitor of acetyl cholinesterase used to treat mild to moderate dementia of the Alzheimer type) was approaching launch in the UK a local group was convened to scrutinize all the available published evidence, background information and unpublished evidence made available by the manufacturer. This group comprised clinicians from general practice, geratology and old age psychiatry, the pharmaceutical adviser to the health authority, a clinical pharmacologist, and a representative from the local Alzheimer's Disease Society. The forum discussed the information presented to it by this local group and considered it under the following headings:

The issue

Alzheimer's disease is a common condition (5000 patients in Oxfordshire) which causes much distress and imposes very significant burdens on patients, their carers, the NHS and social services.

Evidence on effectiveness

One clinical trial (Phase II) had been published at the time of launch, and limited data from an additional randomized double-blind placebo-controlled trial and an open-label extension study were made available to us by the manufacturer. Donepezil (10mg) produced a mean changed in the ADAS-cog (a scoring system specifically developed and validated for quantifying cognitive impairment in Alzheimer's disease) score of 2.88 points (on a 70-point scale) compared with placebo after 24 weeks of treatment. There was no evidence that donepezil improved the quality of life of patients with mild to moderate Alzheimer's disease nor that it increased the likelihood of remaining independent for longer. Donepezil does not affect the underlying disease process.

Value and equity

The patient group and their carers have high need. Donepezil costs around £1000 per annum per patient, to which must also be added the costs of screening patients to identify those who most clearly fit the population studied in clinical trials. Each patient gains three to six months of slightly improved cognition.

Patient choice

Many patients and their carers had expressed a wish to receive donepezil. There was great awareness in the media of the drug launch although the Alzheimer's Disease Society had presented a balanced approach to the product.

Priority

The local group who evaluated the evidence felt that donepezil was of low priority and recommended that it should not be part of normal NHS care and that more information was required.

Decision

The priorities forum agreed with the local group that donepezil was of lower priority than other service pressures not currently funded. The cost for an uncertain but small gain was too great even taking into account the high needs of this group of patients. It was felt that with other new agents in development for Alzheimer's disease, it would be advisable to organize the rather fragmented service for patients with Alzheimer's disease and their carers in order to be able to implement any significant advances effectively in the future.

Conclusion

The forum issued a policy statement (see Box 18.1). When further information and comment was published over the next year this statement was discussed again, but no change was made and the policy was still effective at the beginning of 1999.

Local vs national guidance

Subsequently the Standing Medical Advisory Committee issued a statement on donepezil prefaced by the following general principle: 'Resources should not be diverted to treatments whose clinical benefit and cost-effectiveness is not yet proven.' This statement goes on to say, 'There are currently few published data from primary research on donepezil.' Despite this apparent fulfilment of its own criteria for not diverting resources to donepezil (and there are certainly none lying around waiting to be allocated), the SMAC statement went on to say,

> Where physicians consider that prescription of the drug is justifiable, they should ensure that treatment is carefully targeted and monitored so that patients receive the most benefit from

Box 18.1   Policy statement, July 1997

Donepezil is a new drug licensed for the treatment of mild to moderate dementia in Alzheimer's disease. Current evidence indicates that donepezil produces a modest improvement in cognition, equivalent to 'turning the clock back' by some 3 to 6 months. The benefits are small and the published and accessible unpublished evidence indicates that the drug produces on average an improvement of 3.2 points on a 70-point cognitive scale (ADAS-cog) over 12 weeks. This effect does not increase with time and after the initial improvement the drug does not affect the progression of cognitive decline. There is no evidence to suggest that a sub group of patients is likely to gain significantly greater benefit. (A more detailed assessment of donepezil has been published in Bandolier 40: Vol 4: p. 2–3).

The diagnosis of Alzheimer's disease requires specialist screening and skills, currently mainly provided by the departments of old age psychiatry and geratology. A local expert committee met in April 1997 to assess donepezil and advise the Priorities Forum, and concluded that 'on the evidence so far available on the efficacy and on the cost-effectiveness of donepezil it would not be justifiable to fund its prescription as part of normal NHS care'.

Oxfordshire Health Authority considers donepezil to be of low priority and will not make extra provision to purchase it. Neither will it make available increased funding to screen patients for consideration of treatment with donepezil. Although there is no regulation preventing GPs from prescribing donepezil, Oxfordshire Health Authority's advice is that they should not do so, and no allowance will be made in GP or hospital drug budgets for donepezil.

available resources. The introduction of this treatment should therefore involve accurate diagnosis and systematic monitoring. The variation in response shown to donepezil in clinical research makes pre-treatment selection difficult.

Although SMAC went some way towards identifying these very real concerns with donepezil, by failing to recommend that no resources were diverted to donepezil it ensured that yet again local decisions on priorities have to be made, and local groups need to collate, evaluate and interpret the data and set up systems which fulfil the requirements of 'due process' in local priority setting. It remains to be seen if the national guidance which is promised from the National Institute for Clinical Excellence will be more robust and will help to remove some of the inequities which inevitably arise from local rationing decisions.

THE FUTURE

While the origins of the Priorities Forum lay in the market reforms of the early 1990s, its future in the new millennium lies in cooperation within the locally disparate and diverging system created by the emergence of Primary Care Groups and Trusts. We believe that whatever national guidance is given there will remain a need to discuss and agree clinical priorities across the health care system. Increasingly, the need will exist to consider relative investment between prevention, treatment and care within the National Service Frameworks and to prioritize both health and health care within the Health Improvement Programme. The Priorities Forum will need to address these changes and involve the public increasingly in open and frank discussion about what is and what is not available on the NHS.

19

WHEN SENTIMENTS RUN HIGH: THE DI BELLA CASE AND OTHERS

Silvio Garattini and Vittorio Bertelè

Evidence-based medicine needs to prove that all remedies for the treatment of a disease have a favourable ratio between benefit and risk for the patient. Benefit means a therapeutic effect, essentially a decrease in morbidity and/or mortality. With the advent of national health services, medicines are required not only to be active but also to have a good cost–benefit ratio. With limited financial resources it is important to achieve the best result with the minimum possible expenditure (Maynard 1997). Though this rational approach is accepted in principle, emotions sometimes gain the upper hand and the irrational predominates under pressure from the public, which in turn is influenced by the mass media. This chapter looks at how the public reacts to information about treatments. Several examples will be discussed, in particular the Di Bella case in Italy.

BEFORE DRUG APPROVAL: THE CASE OF ENDOSTATIN AND ANGIOSTATIN

Angiostatin and endostatin are two peptides with anti-angiogenic activity. They reduce tumour growth and dissemination by cutting the blood supply through destruction of newly formed vessels. The results of investigations over 20 years were published in 1997 in *Nature*, an international scientific journal (Boehm *et al.* 1997), without much publicity in the lay press. Several months later Gina Kolada, a *New York Times* journalist, wrote a long article about this 'discovery', which was the starting point for unprecedented interest from the media. The conclusions were very emphatic, particularly when a couple of Nobel prize winners acknowledged this discovery was crucial for the cure of cancer. Although the comments by Judah Folkman, the author of the discovery, were extremely cautious and conservative, many patients wanted the product. However, it was not yet available because no experiments had been carried out on humans.

This report created the hope that anti-angiogenic agents might be enough on their own to cure cancer. People working in the field gained sudden fame; companies announced a number of drugs under study; the US National Cancer Institute expressed interest in the field and the Food and Drug Administration (FDA) authorized Phase 1 trials to begin the following year. Hopes were raised in a number of patients and their families and for several weeks considerable attention was focused on this topic, despite the fact that there was no specific reason for selecting this particular approach to cancer therapy rather than others.

DURING THE PROCESS OF DRUG APPROVAL: THE CASE OF INTERFERON ß

After the publication of an abstract and two articles in *Neurology* (IFNB Multiple Sclerosis Study Group 1993; IFNB Multiple Sclerosis Study Group and the University of British Columbia MS/MRI Analysis Group 1995) Interferon ß (IFN-ß) was perceived by the public as the first effective drug for multiple sclerosis, a relatively rare neurological disease which progresses to severe disability. This information triggered an explosion of requests for rapid authorization from the public and the mass media, with the support of neurology societies and national and international associations of patients with multiple sclerosis.

The drug was considered effective, not for slowing the disability but for preventing about one-third of the exacerbations during the phase called 'relapsing–remitting' disease, and had been approved before by the FDA and then by the European Medicines Evaluation Agency (EMEA) on 12 July 1995. The results of the study were in fact not sufficient to qualify the drug as effective. The number of patients, the design and the criteria used to calculate the outcome were all criticized in the European Public Assessment Report (EPAR) of Betaferon, the proprietary product containing Interferon ß. It is interesting to read the conclusion: 'Because of the significant unmet clinical need for specific treatment of multiple sclerosis, the Betaferon application containing results from two pivotal studies with 372 patients was accepted.'

The number of patients was in fact small at the beginning in the three-arm study (placebo, 123; IFN-ß 1.6 M 125; IFN-ß 8 M 124) and it further decreased because of the number of drop-outs, which reached around 25 per cent after two years, 30 per cent after three years and more than 50 per cent after four years. It is interesting that drop-outs were similar in the three groups. Analysis at five years was done on a total of 166 patients out of the 372 included at the beginning. The annual exacerbation rate was 1.44 for the placebo and 0.96 for the active dose of IFN-ß (8 M) at the end of the first year; the difference decreased after the second year and was no longer statistically significant up to the fifth year. The number of exacerbation-free patients was in favour of IFN-ß only at the second year but not for the other four years. Even these differences could be questioned because they were not analysed on an 'intention-to-treat' basis and the definition of exacerbation excluded those with fever, thus favouring IFN-ß which induces fever which may be concomitant to a relapse. In addition, the duration of relapses was not considered. No effect was observed on the progression of disability, the only parameter that is important for patients.

To avoid one exacerbation, 208 patients must be treated for one year with the approved product. It has been calculated that to avoid one exacerbation the cost of the drug is up to US $ 33,200 in the first year, but the gradual loss of activity means it rises by the 5th year to US $ 71,820. Exacerbations are usually treated with glucocorticosteroids, which may cost US $ 75. Treatment with IFN-β led to a reduction of 127 days in hospital stays during the first three years compared to placebo. A crude calculation indicates that to avoid one day in hospital IFN-β treatment costs about US $ 39,000.

Despite these considerations, annual sales of IFN-β in Italy reached a total of about US $ 60 million in 1997, a quarter of which was for patients with multiple sclerosis.

AFTER DRUG APPROVAL: THE VIAGRA CASE

Viagra is the proprietary name of sildenafil, a chemical which inhibits the enzyme phosphodiesterase 5, that inactivates cyclic guanosine monophosphate (cGMP). This biochemical effect is considered the cause of the relaxation (vasodilation) of the corpora cavernosa which sustains penile erection. Sildenafil is given by the oral route at the dose of 25–100 mg about one hour before sexual activity. About 50 per cent of the patients, compared to 9 per cent with placebo, improved and maintained their erection. However, the studies were limited to 12 weeks' treatment.

The effect of this drug is far from 'magic'. It was less effective in patients over 65 years of age than in younger ones; in cases of severe erectile dysfunction its efficacy was low; patients with radical prostatectomy produced less response than non-prostatectomized patients; psychogenic erectile dysfunctions improved more than patients with mixed etiology or organic dysfunctions. Significant, however, is the observation that sildenafil was better than placebo in subjects with spinal cord injury or transection while diabetics responded less than the broad-spectrum population.

The beneficial effects of sildenafil must be measured against its safety profile. Approval was based on the pooled data of 3003 sildenafil-treated patients vs 1832 placebo-treated. Adverse events were reported in 37 per cent of sildenafil-treated patients and 9 per cent of those given placebo; 17 per cent of the drug-treated patients experienced cardiovascular adverse events (4.8 per cent with placebo), mostly related to vasodilation. Headache, abnormal vision, dyspepsia, myalgia and rare cases of priapism complete the spectrum of adverse effects. As of August 1998 there have been 69 deaths in the USA of men taking sildenafil.

There are several contraindications for sildenafil, including the co-administration of nitric oxide donors or nitrates. In addition the drug should not be given to patients excluded from the clinical studies for severe hepatic impairment, hypotension, recent history of stroke or myocardial infarction, unstable angina, or degenerative retinal disorders. The drug must not be used by people under 18 years of age or by women.

Despite these limitations the approval of the drug in the USA and in Europe (July 1998) was followed by extensive press, radio and television coverage. In most cases the articles were enthusiastic and uncritical. Sildenafil was touted as the drug to improve sexual activity, without explaining that this effect refers to patients with chronic erectile dysfunction and not normal people with occasional dysfunction. The risks were underestimated in respect to the benefit; the idea that only a certain percentage of patients respond to the treatment was overlooked. In general the drug was presented as an aphrodisiac, whereas in reality to be effective it requires appropriate sexual desire and stimulation. Some of the television programmes reported the experiences of well-known personalities who had tried the drug, and its successful use in women was also described.

Interest in the drug – certainly exceeding real needs – is reflected by the sales in the USA. With its projected US $ 1 billion sales per year sildenafil is being sold at its launch more than any other drug in the history of the pharmaceutical market. Clearly emotions are obscuring any rational approach. It is to be hoped that the drug will not be reimbursed by national health services, otherwise a large proportion of pharmaceutical resources will be diverted from more important needs.

WITHOUT ANY DRUG APPROVAL: THE DI BELLA CASE

Almost everybody in Italy by now has heard about somatostatin, an ingredient present in a cocktail of drugs purported by the 86-year-old Professor Luigi Di Bella to be effective in curing almost 100 per cent of cancers as well as multiple sclerosis, Alzheimer's disease, and retinitis pigmentosa. Although reports of miraculous anti-cancer agents crop up frequently, in this case the Italians experienced an unprecedented reaction which created the illusion that the battle against cancer had been won for ever.

The story of Di Bella's 'discovery' started several years ago when he began to treat cancer patients in his home. An organization of patients (ANAN), who had apparently benefited from Di Bella's therapy, attracted the interest of the media when they asked the Italian National Health Services to pay for the therapy. Public interest grew when members of ANAN demonstrated in front of the Department of Health and a judge from Puglia, a region in Southern Italy, followed by several other judges in other Italian regions, obliged the local branch of the National Health Services to supply somatostatin free of charge to a cancer patient for whom a physician had prescribed the therapy.

Somatostatin is an expensive drug in Italy: three mg per day – the usual dose – costs about 5,435 ECU a month. The judges' initiative created a debate among politicians, and the right-wing party, Alleanza Nazionale, took a clear position in favour of Di Bella. Since December 1997, stories have flooded the Italian press. Television, radio, newspapers and magazines devoted considerable space to an old man who had developed a 'cure' for cancer after years of personal effort. According to the press he did it all without asking patients for money, and he was persecuted by the academic world because he worked against the interests of the powerful multi-national pharmaceutical giants. Unfortunately, the academic world – with few exceptions – particularly oncologists, did not or could not take a strong opposing position for fear of alienating the public, and especially their patients. Additionally, the press proved particularly impermeable to any information that diminished Di Bella's prestige. Only patients who expressed a positive opinion were interviewed, judges who reached a negative opinion about the compulsory payment by the National Health Service were not mentioned and science writers were not allowed to express their views.

Patients are the obvious victims of this 'Italian saga' as some have stopped conventional treatments to devote themselves to Di Bella's therapy. Confusion and desperation reached a peak when it became clear that supplies of somatostatin were inadequate for the large number of patients demanding the drug. Fortunately the Minister of Health very strongly defended the principle that only proven effective drugs could be reimbursed by the National Health Service, despite protests from Parliament and the Senate.

At this point it may be necessary to describe Di Bella's therapy. The cocktail includes not only somatostatin – or octreotide, a longer-acting derivative – but also melatonin, bromocryptine, a mixture of vitamins, adrenocorticotropic hormone and usually 100 mg oral cyclophosphamide, a low dose of a chemotherapeutic agent employed in several polychemotherapy regimens for different cancers.

Discovered in 1993, somatostatin inhibits the release of growth hormone and is indicated in the treatment of acromegaly. Somatostatin and its analogue octreotide are also indicated for the relief of symptoms associated with relatively rare tumours such as carcinoids, VIPomas and glucagonomas. Bromocryptine is a weak inhibitor of growth hormone release, but is used mostly as a dopaminergic agonist for the treatment of prolactinomas and Parkinson's disease. Melatonin is not yet marketed in Italy, but it has no specific indication with the possible exception of sleep disturbances due to jet-lag. The other components of the cocktail are not worth noting.

One searches in vain for scientific publications by Di Bella in the field of oncology or on the efficacy of his therapy. The one exception is an abstract from a meeting held in Athens by the pharmaceutical company producing somatostatin. There, Di Bella qualitatively described his therapy but stated that somatostatin was

useless in patients with advanced cancers. In the midst of the tur-
moil of protest and requests by Di Bella fans, the Italian government decided to organize a Phase II clinical trial. Because of the
interchanges between politicians and oncologists, the trial was
designed to include ten protocols and – with the so-called obser-
vational study – a total of about 3000 patients. A Phase II trial usually starts with 30–50 patients. What should have been done was
first to analyse the clinical dossiers of the patients treated by Di
Bella and select the tumour which was apparently most sensitive.
This would have resulted in a real Phase II study and avoided
exposing so many patients to a therapy with no scientific basis.

In the meantime the Italian Constitutional Court stated that
people with low income could be given the Di Bella therapy free of
charge at the expense of the National Health Service. To finance
this unexpected expense Parliament decided to raise the 'ticket' for
drug prescription by about 6 per cent. Ironically, approval of this
decree arrived a few hours before the presentation of the results of
the four protocols that concluded the Phase II trial. In summary the
results were as follows:

- 34 patients with metastatic mammary cancer not eligible for
  chemotherapy or hormonal therapy: 15 patients died; no evidence of response;
- 34 patients with advanced colorectal carcinoma: 7 patients died;
  no evidence of response;
- 34 patients with carcinoma of cervico-facial oesophagus: 15
  patients died; no evidence of response;
- 34 patients with different tumours in a terminal phase: 20 patients
  died; no evidence of response.

While negative results were expected, it was certainly a surprise –
considering Di Bella's assurances about the perfect safety of the
treatment – to see the number of adverse events: 35–65 per cent
according to the protocol.

Considering the four protocols together, at the end of treatment
75 per cent of the patients had died or were in a condition of tumour
progression, 13 per cent had discontinued the treatment spon-
taneously or because of the toxicity, 9 per cent remained stable and
3 per cent were not evaluable. It should be noted that in the
multicentre trial about 40 per cent of the patients were in moderate
conditions.

Obviously Di Bella and his supporters rejected these results,
insisting the trials had not been conducted according to his protocol.
The cost of the Di Bella case is not exactly known, but considering

the costs of the drugs and staffing and organizing the clinical trials, it may run close to 50 billion Italian lire (about US $ 29 million). It is sad to note that Italian scientists working on cancer did not receive any funds for 1998 because financial restrictions meant it was not possible to provide the US $ 14 million required for the Research National Council project on cancer.

CONCLUSION

The cases presented here have a common denominator: an excess of confidence in the effectiveness of drugs for the solution of both severe and minor problems. These cases are obviously extreme but they are part of a pharmaco-centric culture that delegates the solution of medical problems only to medicines.

There is no doubt that the mass media have most of the responsibility for creating illusions for patients who are the innocent victims of a race to publicize results and expectations. In addition, in many cases there are formidable financial interests behind the scenes. However, it is also surprising how little influence is exerted by scientific leaders and societies and, more generally, by the medical world, on information to the public. This situation leads in most cases to an undue financial burden on individuals and the national health services.

There are no magic solutions, but obviously the problem must be discussed if appropriate action is to be taken. First of all it is important not only to improve the level of scientific understanding among opinion leaders and the press, but also to underline their responsibilities to patients. Second, we must strengthen the action of the scientific and medical communities. A permanent national or international body should be set up to react very rapidly with clear and credible information any time there is a tendency to spread distorted news about new therapeutic interventions. Third, the public's knowledge needs to be improved. Perhaps our schools are not geared to conveying simple scientific information such as the concepts of probability and risk, the difficulty of establishing the relation between cause and effect, and the principles that must be respected before concluding that a drug is effective for a given disease.

These inadequacies, which are certainly not easy to overcome, will be responsible for the next Di Bella case that may arise in Italy or anywhere else. For this reason measures should be taken on a European rather than a national scale, mobilizing and strengthening the forces already available.

20

INCREASING DEMAND FOR ACCOUNTABILITY: IS THERE A PROFESSIONAL RESPONSE?

Ole Frithjof Norheim

The concept of deliberative democracy, the idea that legitimate democracy issues from the public deliberation of citizens, is emerging as an underlying idea of much of the recent development in the theory of medical rationing (Eddy 1990a; Klein 1993a; Ezekiel and Ezekiel 1996; New 1996; Thompson 1996; Daniels and Sabin 1997; Elster, 1998). One important element in that concept is the idea of public accountability. Simplifying the debate, we may say that rationing decisions satisfy the requirements of public accountability if all relevant reasons for the decisions are given by those responsible for it to those who are affected by it (Gutman and Thompson 1996). This – in one sense rather narrow – definition refers to a concept of rationing which needs a few comments.

RATIONING

Richard Smith's recent comment about the UK National Health Service (NHS) applies fairly well in many countries. I take it as the point of departure for this chapter:

> The fiction of the NHS, encouraged by this government and the last, is that the NHS can provide a comprehensive, high quality service that is free at the point of delivery and covers everybody. The reality, well recognised by most of those

working in the service, is that health systems cannot meet all four principles.

(Smith 1998: 760)

Assuming that Smith is correct, this makes rationing a topic especially appropriate for the theory of deliberative democracy.

This chapter defines rationing as the withholding of potentially beneficial health care through financial or organizational features of the health care system in question. Some reserve the concept 'rationing' for micro mechanisms and decisions that affect individual patients (second-order decisions) and 'priority setting' for macro decisions concerning the capacity of a given service for a given group (first-order decisions) (Klein 1995). In my view, this is a useful distinction. This chapter, however, concentrates on issues at the meso or intermediate level where formal and informal rules guide decisions concerning groups of patients. The difference between rationing and priority setting is not clear cut. Here the term rationing is also used for decision making at the meso level.

The professional response to rationing

In the literature on priority setting in health care, the claim that services with no documented effect can legitimately be withheld is one of its basic assumptions. The methods of evidence-based medicine (EBM) therefore seem to be natural building blocks in any professional response to the problem of who should have what kind of health care. According to Sackett *et al.*'s definition: 'evidence-based medicine is the process of systematically finding, appraising, and using contemporaneous research findings as the basis for clinical decisions' (Sackett *et al.* 1997). The aim is to make the best choice for the patient on the basis of available evidence. The following example illuminates how the methods of EBM can be seen as a response to the demands for accountability.

Outcome and costs of lowering cholesterol concentration with statins in patients with and without pre-existing coronary heart disease

Consider the following case: a 56-year-old man with no known coronary heart disease, occasional chest pain, and a serum-cholesterol of 7.0 mmol/l measured after diet and lifestyle changes, approaches the doctor and asks for advice on whether there are any drugs that could reduce his health risks.

The modern, professionally accountable doctor would search for the best available evidence about any treatment that would effectively and safely reduce the health risks of this person. A systematic literature search according to the principles of evidence-based medicine would probably result in a large set of publications of well-designed clinical trials.

Two major randomized clinical trials satisfying the stringent criteria of validity, importance and applicability are the Scandinavian Simvastatin Survival Study (the 4S-study) published in the *Lancet* in 1994 and the West of Scotland Coronary Prevention Study published in the *New England Journal of Medicine* in 1995 (Scandinavian Simvastatin Group 1994; Sheperd *et al.* 1995). The first study provides robust and valid evidence for the effectiveness of lowering cholesterol concentration with Simvastatin in patients aged 35–70 years who have a history of coronary heart disease and a serum cholesterol concentration > 5.4 mmol/l. The second study, although more controversial, provides evidence for the effect and safety of Pravastatin in men aged 45–64 years with no history of coronary heart disease and a cholesterol concentration of > 6.4 mmol/l.

After consulting the evidence, the next step for our doctor would be to perform certain diagnostic tests with the aim of finding out whether the patient's chest pain could be attributed to coronary heart disease. An affirmative answer would locate our patient in a different diagnostic group than a negative answer. After performing the diagnostic tests, the chest pain is diagnosed as oesophagitis, not angina pectoris.

The underlying clinical reasoning in this case is the following. Based on the available evidence and information about certain characteristics of patients (age, sex and pre-existing coronary heart disease), it is possible to classify those with high cholesterol concentrations into different risk and benefit groups. Let us call them priority groups (see Table 20.1).

Considering the characteristics of our patient (a man aged 56 with no history of coronary heart disease and a cholesterol concentration of 7.0 mmol/l) the physician would classify him as Group 3. His estimated five-year risk of death from coronary heart disease or a non-fatal myocardial infarction would be 7.9 per cent, and the expected benefit would be an absolute risk reduction of 2.4 per cent to 5.5 per cent. This is reported as a relative risk reduction of 31 per cent (CI 17–43) (Sheperd *et al.* 1995). Numbers needed to treat to prevent one such event would be 45.

Table 20.1 Priority groups: classification of patients with moderate to high cholesterol concentration according to age, sex and pre-existing coronary heart disease

---

Group 1 – men aged 45–64 and women aged 55–64 with previous myocardial infarction and a cholesterol concentration > 5.4 mmol/l

Group 2 – men aged 45–64 and women aged 55–64 with angina and a cholesterol concentration > 5.4 mmol/l

Group 3 – men aged 55–64 with no history of coronary heart disease and cholesterol > 6.5 mmol/l

Group 4 – women aged 45–54 with angina or previous myocardial infarction and a cholesterol concentration > 5.4 mmol/l

Group 5 – men aged 45–54 with no history of coronary heart disease and cholesterol > 6.5 mmol/l

---

Source: Based on Pharoah and Hollingworth 1996

Clinical choice: evidence, rules and values

The doctor's conclusion – based on the best evidence, considering the medical and prognostic characteristics of the patient in front of him, and also being attentive to his preferences after having informed him about all the facts – is that he should prescribe Pravastatin or a similar drug.

Now, both our patient and the doctor live in Norway. In this public health care system, funded mainly by tax revenues, there are some restrictions on reimbursement of service expenditures. The guidelines regulating reimbursement for expensive long-term drug therapy have set the cut-off point for patients without coronary heart disease and high cholesterol levels at > 8.0 mmol/l (the drug must also be prescribed by a specialist) (Sosialdepartementet 1998). This patient does not qualify for reimbursement of the treatment costs. So all beneficial treatment is not free at the point of delivery.

Although the rationale for the cut-off point of 8.0 mmol/l is not given explicitly by the Department of Health, our modern doctor will assume that it has something to do with costs (or alternatively, delay in the response to new evidence). There is, however, nowhere he can search for the rationale of this specific decision.

Instead he performs a search for valid, important and applicable cost-effectiveness studies, again according to the criteria of EBM. He ends up with, among others, the Pharoah and Hollingworth study published in the *BMJ* in 1996 (Pharoah and Hollingworth 1996). This is a model-based cost-effectiveness study citing only evidence that would meet the criteria of validity, importance and applicability considered earlier. The study analyses the cost implications of expanding indications to include various risk groups of patients with high cholesterol for the population of Cambridge and Huntingdon Health Commission.

The study shows that if all risk groups (1–5 in Table 20.1) were included in Cambridge and Huntingdon Health Commission, a population with 95,800 resident men and women aged 45–64 years, net costs over a 10-year period would amount to more than £88 million. Total life years saved would be 967. Including Risk Group 1–3 (including the patient in our example and all others with equal or greater expected benefits) would save 761 life years at a net cost of approximately £38 million.

Although public costs are considerable, the Norwegian doctor knows that the patient will certainly complain if not given reimbursement because his long-term costs are fairly expensive and the rationale for the cut-off point is not clear to him. The patient expects long-term treatment with costly, beneficial and safe drugs to be reimbursed from Social Insurance if prescribed by a competent doctor.

The Office of National Insurance, the Department of Health and the Office of Drug Approval formulate the regulations. In controversial cases, the final decision rests with the Parliament. In this special case the regulations date back to 1994. They have not been adjusted according to new evidence published, and the health authorities give no reasons for the restrictive rules.

The doctor would, in his meeting with this patient, face at least three options:

- *Non-rationing:* he could prescribe the drug and let the public system cover most of the expenses. No one would control or demand a rationale for his decision.
- *Implicit rationing:* he could tell the patient that the benefits of the treatment are non-existent or marginal, the evidence uncertain and that his advice would be not to take the drug.
- *Explicit rationing:* he could prescribe the drug, explain the rules of reimbursement, inform him about the public cost and let the patient cover the expenses.

The choice is left to the doctor's discretion. I shall not attempt to describe what Norwegian doctors do. It is the structure of the choice situation that is of interest. The incentive structure in such cases is well known. The existence of third-party payers tends to

favour the first solution: non-rationing. Many responsible physicians will, at least according to my experience from Norway, go for
the second solution: implicit rationing. Let us now examine how
both choices violate, in different ways, the requirements of accountability.

THE REQUIREMENTS OF PUBLIC
ACCOUNTABILITY

Rationing choices satisfy the requirements of public accountability
if all the relevant reasons are given by those responsible for the
decision to those who are affected by it.

Relevant reasons

In our context three groups of reasons are relevant for withholding
a given service:

- medical reasons;
- economic or political reasons; and
- normative reasons.

More needs to be said about the third kind of reasons.

Normative reasons

If resources are scarce, normative reasons can be given for not providing an intervention that is potentially beneficial. Such reasons
can be that:

- the expected outcome is not important enough;
- the burden of disease (if untreated) is not important enough for
  public concern;
- the costs are too high compared to the benefit;
- other patients have stronger claims on scarce resources;
- the costs can be borne by the patient him- or herself;
- evidence is inconclusive.

These reasons are normative in the sense that they require the
patient (and his or her physician) to give up a benefit by an appeal
to some notion of what is the right or the good thing to do. In the
case of cholesterol-lowering drugs for patients without pre-existing coronary heart disease, several of these arguments could be

advanced to justify exclusion of this low-benefit group. I believe also that the majority of the population would accept these reasons. The point is, however, that for our patient, these arguments have never been provided. It is therefore impossible for him to assess the legitimacy of the rationing decision by which he is affected.

By whom, to whom?

Who is responsible for providing the explanations that are required for public accountability? There is no easy answer to this. In principle we could argue that politicians and administrative managers responsible for first-order decisions should provide the economic or political reasons for their decisions. Physicians making second-order decisions should give the medical reasons for their recommendations. But who should give the normative reasons? In my view, these reasons cannot be separated from either the medical or the economic reasons. The normative reasons should therefore be provided by both groups of decision makers to those affected by them. Those affected include not only patients but also citizens with an interest in the public use of resources. Patients and citizens are related to each other through a net of relationships where other groups (such as various medical specialties, patients' organizations, providers, health authorities and politicians) represent or oppose their interests. Decisions and their justification should be accessible to all these groups. Accountability requires institutions to ensure that reasons for rationing are accessible to all affected parties.

Summing up the dilemma about whether our modern professional physician should choose non-rationing, implicit rationing or explicit rationing, we can conclude that non-rationing would violate normative accountability, but not the norms of evidence-based medicine. There are medical reasons to prescribe the drug, and since the health authorities do not openly endorse rationing, why should he bother? Implicit rationing, on the other hand, would violate medical accountability, but could help contain costs and probably redirect scarce resources toward more needy patients. What we have here are different systems of norms: the 'medical' norm that all beneficial interventions should be provided free of charge (the ideal of Archie Cochrane, see Maynard 1997), and the norms of public officials that require consideration of costs and competing needs within resource constraints (Drummond 1998).

OBSTACLES TO PUBLIC ACCOUNTABILITY

Let us examine in more detail the obstacles to public accountability. Should not the responsible, accountable physician reject non-rationing and implicit rationing?

First, the profession has few economic incentives for explicit rationing. Second, the profession has clear interests in insisting on the 'art' of medical judgement – preserving professional autonomy – instead of following strict administrative rules or 'cook-book medicine'. Third, there are personal mechanisms that create incentives to comply with patients' preferences. Moreover, explicit rationing is problematic without backing from health authorities. Physicians are meeting patients face-to-face on a daily basis. We cannot expect doctors to be willing to take the blame for those decisions when the political system is upholding the fiction that the system can provide 'a comprehensive, high quality service that is free at the point of delivery and covers everybody'. In sum, neither incentives nor support from health authorities are in place to encourage the profession to ration explicitly at the micro level.

There are, on the other hand, plausible grounds for the health authorities not to admit that the system is rationing effective interventions. First, the role of the media in such cases should not be underestimated. Few politicians would take part in such self-defeating practices. Second, there is a clear intersection of interests between the government and the medical profession on this question. Implicit rationing preserves professional autonomy *and* reduces blame on the political system (Klein 1993b).

Add to this the organizational features of most health care systems. Decentralization, regionalization and differentiation into various administrative levels uphold a system of divided responsibility that renders economic and political accountability almost impossible.

Next, unlike the standard of validity in evidence-based medicine, there exists no theoretical or publicly approved standard of acceptable reasons for limit-setting decisions (New 1996). This stems partly from the special characteristics of health services. The benefits of health care involve risks and risk reduction that are perceived and valued differently. Is the risk reduction of 2.4 per cent over five years for the patient in our example important or not? Compared to what? We lack common standards and concepts to comprehend such risks. The expected benefits of new technologies and new drugs are difficult to measure and, some argue, impossible to compare. Observe also that normative reasons include contested judgements about the value of outcomes, the burden of disease or the strength of claims. They refer to notions such as cost and cost-effectiveness, and they refer to fundamental normative values such as equality, fairness in distribution or maximization of health benefits.

Another obstacle to accountability is asymmetry of information, the mechanism said to create market failure. According to standard health economic theory, asymmetric information between the profession and consumers makes it difficult to develop and maintain consistent preferences about which services should be purchased (Arrow 1963b). The same mechanism makes it difficult for citizens to form consistent interests that could influence deliberative priority setting in a sensible way. Asymmetric information creates 'democratic failure'. The fear of this might explain the scepticism about involving the public through explicit rationing.

SHOULD CLINICIANS TAKE THE LEAD?

When rationing is the main issue, there are few arenas in which 'evidence can be tested against arguments' and against conflicting systems of norms (Klein 1993a). Rationing seems to be the non-existing health policy question. Reasons for rationing cannot therefore be scrutinized, criticized or revised in public.

To establish an institution to coordinate such activity would probably be costly. It would require medical and other expertise that could better be used elsewhere and would increase the number of people employed in management. It could increase bureaucracy, and we know little about whether the results could be implemented (Mechanic 1995).

What clinicians can do is build on their existing institutions and promote publicity and transparency at the meso level, for instance in the development of clinical guidelines (Hayward *et al.* 1995; Wilson *et al.* 1995). The medical profession needs to adopt an attitude as creative, innovative and enthusiastic as the EBM movement. It should, however, be guided by the idea of public involvement and accountability – not just medical rationality (Daniels and Sabin 1995).

WHAT CAN WE LEARN FROM EBM?

The first section showed how medical reasons could be based on the systematic assessment of evidence. That is not to say that the evidence *is* the truth. There is in the scientific community a set of institutions and procedures that ensure that evidence is produced and can be relied upon – at least provisionally until new evidence challenges our previous beliefs. These institutions and procedures (the educational system, university hospitals, scientific journals, conferences, etc.) are far from faultless, but they are the grounds that traditionally have guaranteed the authority of medical decisions and medical reasons. These institutions:

- rely on procedures that secure the quality of the documentation (peer review, the hierarchy of medical journals, standards of excellence in research);
- encourage publication of methods and results, ensuring that evidence can be scrutinized, challenged and revised;
- foster a continuous debate about the criteria of validity;
- ground the legitimacy of medical judgements.

Evidence-based medicine can be seen as a methodology that makes the scientific norms of the profession explicit, grounds clinical decisions in good medical reasons and clarifies what the standards of good evidence are.

Building upon this approach, for instance in the development of clinical guidelines, the profession could promote publicity and transparency in many ways. A possible checklist is given below:

- specify whether rationing is part of the decision problem;
- identify both medical reasons and normative reasons for the clinical choice in question;
- identify stratified priority groups for the service in question (as in Table 20.1 on the five risk–benefit groups for persons with hypercholesterolemia);
- express the expected benefits in a language that all decision makers and affected parties can comprehend (e.g. numbers needed to treat, absolute risk reduction);
- make the consequences of limit setting explicit for each priority group.

This is not the place to develop these ideas in detail (Norheim 1996). My point is merely to indicate that openness and transparency is possible and could be built into already existing methods for guideline development (Eddy 1990a, 1990b). I believe the long-term impact of openness and transparency cannot be under-estimated. It can reduce asymmetric information and make involvement of the public more realistic. Making rationing choices transparent at the meso level might also reduce the pressures at the micro level and, hopefully, increase pressure at the macro level towards the establishment of procedures and institutions fostering deliberative health politics.

CONCLUSION

I would like to conclude, however, with some sceptical thoughts about the feasibility of the ideal of explicit rationing. The case of cholesterol-lowering drugs has not been handled very well in Norway. This is so despite the fact that funding is centralized and that the cut-off point is defined precisely according to objective criteria (a biochemical test). What about other rationing issues then – such as treatment for mental disorders, the use of hysterectomies, cartilage transplantation for knee disorders, Aricept for Alzheimer's disease or Viagra for erectile dysfunction – where precise criteria for proper inclusion are hard to define, evidence is inconclusive or funding is fragmented? I do not know. A modest conclusion is, however, that we need more public deliberation on these issues, not less.

21

CONCLUSION:
WHERE ARE WE NOW?
Chris Ham and Angela Coulter

The experience and research reported in this book illustrate both the complexity of rationing and the extent of unfinished business. As we noted in the Introduction, setting priorities for health care is not amenable to simple or technical solutions that will resolve the dilemmas that arise once and for all. Rather, rationing is akin to an extended exercise in policy learning, involving trial and error and the adjustment of direction in the light of experience. Debates about health care priorities also exemplify the struggle for power in health systems with a variety of stakeholders seeking to influence decisions while avoiding responsibility and blame when things go wrong. The idea that policy making involves both puzzling about problems and bargaining between different interests is well established in the literature on comparative social policy (Heclo 1974), and much of the work presented here lends support to this thesis.

In this Conclusion, we bring together the main themes from the different chapters, following the same framework as in the Introduction but extending this to identify new issues that emerge from experience. In the process, we seek to distil the most significant lessons that can be drawn from the work done so far in the hope that these lessons will be of use to those responsible for rationing. We also reflect on the implications for researchers into health policy. Analysis of the substance and process of rationing is fertile territory for the exploration of not only the struggle for power between different interests but also the future of democratic deliberation in health care. As many of the contributors have identified these as key issues, we draw on their work to indicate how work on rationing might be taken forward.

LEVELS OF RATIONING

The existence of a number of levels of rationing is amply demonstrated by the contributors to this book. Reshaping priorities on a global level requires concerted action by the international community, a daunting task in view of the difficulties faced within countries. Yet Bryant and Khan have drawn attention to the impact of the global economy and international political tensions on the health of the poorest people in developing countries. Both authors stress the importance of international collaboration in tackling health inequalities and redistribution of resources.

Several authors focus on priority setting at the macro level and report experience from countries where there have been national initiatives. The Nordic countries are of particular interest in this context, having taken the lead at an early stage to establish national committees to advise on what should be done and now revisiting the work of these committees in the light of further experience. Palo describes recent developments in Finland in this regard while Holm offers a comparative overview of Nordic experience. Holm argues on the basis of his overview that macro approaches are entering a second phase in which less emphasis is being placed on the search for technical solutions and greater attention is being given to the process of decision making, a theme to which we return below.

Chinitz and colleagues and Edgar report on developments in Israel and New Zealand respectively. The experience of Israel is important in adding another example to the growing stock of stories about countries that have grasped the nettle of explicit rationing at a macro level. A key lesson here is that the basic health care package was defined both generally and broadly with the government determining the cost of the package. In practice, expenditures have exceeded revenues, leading to financial deficits. This in turn has prompted debate about restricting the coverage of the package to essential services and there have been protests and lobbying by groups who have felt disadvantaged. Political struggles within government have contributed to the complexity of these debates and on the basis of the progress report offered by Chinitz and colleagues the long-term outcome remains uncertain.

Like the Nordic countries, New Zealand has several years' experience of seeking to be more systematic about rationing at a national level. As someone who has been at the heart of this work, Edgar is refreshingly honest in highlighting both achievements and the distance yet to be travelled. The pragmatism of the work of the National Health Committee emerges strongly from her analysis with a focus of effort in areas where the committee felt progress could be made. What is unclear at the end of Edgar's account is how much real influence the committee has had on decision making. In the absence of any formal evaluations, this can only be a matter of speculation but the impression gained from the work done in both New Zealand and other countries that have tried to be systematic about rationing at a macro level is that there is often a gap between the recommendations of national groups and what happens in practice.

The importance of the meso level of rationing is demonstrated in the chapters by Griffiths and colleagues and by Williams and Yeo. The latter authors describe the process of regionalization in the Canadian provinces with the increased responsibility this places on the members of regional boards. Williams and Yeo speculate about the ethical dilemmas this will raise and their concerns are underscored by the experience in an English health authority set out by Griffiths and colleagues. As these authors show, in the United Kingdom the meso level is particularly important and health authorities have a key role at this level in setting priorities. In Oxfordshire, the approach adopted has involved developing a number of principles to guide decision making and refining the process for considering options to generate legitimacy for the choices that are made. As in the work of the National Health Committee in New Zealand, the relative priority attached to different services and involving the public in the process remain important challenges.

Sabin's chapter puts the role of clinicians centre stage and in so doing turns the focus to the micro level. The central issue here, raised by a number of authors, is the potential conflict for clinicians in acting as agents and advocates for individual patients and assuming stewardship for the population as a whole. In the United States the rapid expansion of managed care has pointed up this conflict, particularly when physicians work under budgetary systems that may create an incentive not only to weigh the claims of different patients but also to consider the cost of treatment in relation to the impact on physicians' own incomes. Both Clancy and Danis and Daniels comment on this, with Daniels suggesting a need for managed care organizations to demonstrate that the reimbursement of physicians is compatible with appropriate care.

Sabin's view is that there is no inherent conflict between the physician's love for patients (or in his terms 'fidelity') and population stewardship. In taking this view, he is challenging the argument that making clinicians responsible for rationing is a form of blame diffusion. Indeed, Sabin goes further to argue that doctors are particularly well placed to lead the debate on rationing because of the trust that exists between patients and doctors and the opportunities available to doctors to use their encounters with patients to inform and educate. Drawing on his own experience as a psychiatrist, Sabin shows how a commonsense approach to these issues can work and he argues that politicians need to adopt the same kind of approach at a societal level, given that the days of implicit rationing are over.

TECHNIQUES AND JUDGEMENT

The role of techniques in rationing, especially those drawn from economics, is emphasized in Williams's chapter. Reiterating views expressed over a number of years, Williams argues that effective priority setting requires clarity about objectives, information about costs and outcomes, and the ability to measure performance. Specifically, Williams makes a plea for greater attention to be given to defining and measuring outcomes and 'the adoption of economic appraisal techniques as the standard evaluative method for all health care activities' (p. 19–20). In so doing, Williams is throwing down a challenge to policy makers and others who prefer to muddle through rather than set priorities on an explicit basis. A rather different view is advanced by Klein who draws attention to the shortcomings of technical approaches and emphasizes instead the essentially contested nature of rationing and the role of judgement in making decisions on resource allocation. For Klein the task is less to refine the technical basis of decision making than to construct a process that enables proper debate and discussion to occur. In his terms, this debate 'cannot be resolved by an appeal to science . . . Hence the crucial importance of getting the institutional setting of the debate right' (p. 21). As we discuss below, this is a theme addressed by several other authors.

Klein's arguments are reinforced by experience from the Nordic countries as reported by Holm. As he describes, the first phase of work on rationing in these countries was characterized by 'a search for priority setting systems that, through a complete and non-contradictory set of rational decision rules, could tell the decision maker precisely how a given service should be prioritised vis-à-vis other services' (p. 31).

Later work demonstrated the difficulty of discovering such rules. To quote Holm again, it was recognized that

> we cannot reduce the goal of a public health care system of the Nordic type to only one thing. A public health care system is not there simply to maximize the amount of health in society (however we choose to measure health). It is not there merely to treat disease (however we choose to define disease). It is not there solely to meet health care needs (however we choose to define health care needs). And it is not there to ensure equality in health status (however we choose to conceptualize equality). The goal of a public health care system is a complex composite of a range of goals . . . This means that it becomes impossible to use a simple maximizing algorithm as a basis for the priority setting system (pp. 31–2).

At the micro level, Dennett and Parry report from New Zealand on the impact of applying techniques in the form of objective scoring systems to establish priorities for patients waiting for surgery. In this case, the techniques were not well designed and produced results which were both anomalous and unacceptable to clinicians. Dennett and Parry argue that this was because clinicians were not involved adequately in the development of scoring systems and the effect was to discriminate against patients who could benefit from surgery. Their conclusion that linear analogue scores based on clinical judgement are preferable to apparently objective and scientific techniques stands as a cautionary tale. As such, it reinforces the warning from Mullen that the techniques that are used in rationing must be rigorous and appropriate to the purpose.

Yet if techniques cannot provide the holy grail sought by some, they nevertheless have a contribution to make in informing debate about rationing decisions. This is demonstrated by several authors who show how both quantitative and qualitative analysis can provide an input to decision making. This is a clear message from Edgar's account of experience in New Zealand and suggests that the debate between Williams and Klein may be drawn too starkly. There is no inherent conflict between, on the one hand, action to provide more and better information on the costs and outcomes of different interventions and, on the other, work to strengthen the processes for debating that information and arriving at judgements on priorities. To be sure, the relative importance attached to these activities is an issue that divides economists and policy analysts but there may be more common ground in this debate than at first appears. As we argue at the end of this chapter, in the next phase of rationing there is a need to go beyond the dichotomies that have polarized debate in this area and seek a new synthesis between different perspectives.

PUBLIC INVOLVEMENT

Several authors comment on public involvement in rationing. While most do so from a position of wanting to encourage the greater involvement of both patients and the public in debates in this field, both Mullen and Coast are more cautious. Mullen points out that

> Concerns about the legitimacy of public involvement relate to the 'representativeness' of those participating, the perceived lack of knowledge of lay people in an area populated by professionals, the risk of populism and even public resistance to being involved in 'rationing'. There is also concern that public participation is being used to compensate for the lack of democracy . . . (pp. 163–4).

She adds that there is a need for methodological rigour in deciding how to involve the public, adding that this is more important when the purpose is to use the results to determine priorities than when the aim is to find a way of allowing the public to take part in the process of decision making. Her review of different methods of public involvement serves as a reminder that there is considerable experience of work in this field and a need to avoid reinventing the wheel.

Coast's arguments are related to the concerns raised by Mullen, in particular to the adverse effects there may be on those who are asked to participate in rationing. Using the language of economics, Coast seeks to explore through interviews with members of the public the extent to which participation may result in disutility. Her findings, although based on a small-scale project, indicate that members of the public are more concerned at denying others treatment than being told that their own care is being rationed. Indeed, the results suggest that the public prefer to know that they are not receiving treatment, a conclusion that supports the arguments advanced by Sabin and other authors for greater openness between doctors and patients and between politicians and the public.

Edgar's account of experience in New Zealand provides a rich source of information about the path taken in that country to engage the public. As she notes, there are many different publics and many different ways of encouraging these publics to participate. The purpose of participation has also varied and 'Objectives have ranged from information sharing and awareness raising, through opinion gathering, to input on specific questions or identification of service priorities' (p. 177).

In the early stages of its work the National Health Committee put the emphasis on explaining why rationing was necessary and using the results of consultation to recommend broad priorities. As its work developed, participation was channelled in a more focused way through lay involvement in consensus panels, guideline development, contested hearings, focus groups and other methods. Despite these efforts, Edgar emphasizes that there is still a long way to go to develop a more informed understanding of rationing, a point echoed by Garattini and Bertele in their account of experience in Italy. The New Zealand work is being taken forward through a consumer training programme in guidelines development which in Edgar's view 'should raise public engagement by several notches' (pp. 188–9).

EXCLUDING SERVICES

The difficulty of excluding services from funding, noted in the Introduction, is supported by a number of contributions. At a macro level, the experience of Israel echoes that of the Netherlands in demonstrating that proposals to restrict the benefits package provoke opposition and more often than not are likely to be defeated. Not only this, but also, as Chinitz and colleagues show, explicit rationing in Israel has resulted in new drugs and services being added to the benefits package. In this sense, the Israel case confirms experience in both Oregon and New Zealand where explicit rationing also had the effect of increasing the scope of services covered (Ham 1998a) and forcing politicians to increase the health care budget. A further similarity with Oregon (although not New Zealand) is that politicians have responded to financial deficits by placing more of the burden on users through co-payments (Ham 1998b) rather than by restricting service coverage.

More generally, the reluctance to rule out whole categories of care may be inferred from the approach taken by committees and expert groups set up to discuss rationing at a macro level and the response of governments to the reports of these groups. As we highlighted in the Introduction, the approach taken in Oregon of defining a list of treatments to be funded is the exception rather than the rule. Both expert groups and politicians have backed off rationing by exclusion both because of the high political costs associated with this approach and because an argument can be made in the case of any treatment suggested for exclusion that some patients will benefit. As a consequence, responsibility for decision making has been passed down to the meso and micro levels where managers and clinicians have had to confront the challenge.

This is clearly demonstrated in Ham's account of the Child B case in the United Kingdom and it is underlined by other authors who note the emphasis placed on clinicians as the ultimate arbiters of who should receive treatment. As Norheim notes, citing Klein, there is an incentive for both politicians and clinicians to avoid explicit rationing because being implicit preserves professional autonomy for clinicians and deflects blame away from politicians. The only rider to add to this is that the collusion between politicians and clinicians to avoid explicitness may break down when financial pressures combined with rising patient demands make implicit decision making too uncomfortable for doctors to sustain. That point may not yet have been reached but in most systems its arrival appears imminent.

The evidence on patient attitudes to the denial of treatment is contradictory. Ham's chapter on the Child B case in the United Kingdom, with its account of a father unwilling to accept the advice of paediatricians and actively seeking further clinical opinions, is reinforced by experience from New Zealand, Israel and Italy. In all of these countries, patients and groups who felt they were being denied treatment were successful in persuading politicians to change their decisions on funding and were not prepared to acquiesce to restrictions on the availability of care. On the other hand, there is the argument of Sabin that patients who understand the reasons for restrictions on services are willing to acquiesce, especially when clinicians give the explanation. Against this, Coast's research indicates that some individuals want information about the denial of treatment to help them accept medical decisions whereas others see access to information as a way of challenging clinical judgements. The existence of the latter group lends support to the argument that the days of deference are coming to an end.

GUIDELINES

The use of guidelines as a tool of rationing is evident in a number of countries. Norheim's example of the part played by guidelines in the prescribing of statins in Norway illustrates both the pitfalls and possibilities of this approach. At one level, guidelines offer the potential to ensure that treatment is provided appropriately and effectively, but at another they risk losing credibility and being bypassed if they are not developed with the support and commitment of clinicians. A similar conclusion is indicated by Dennett and Parry's analysis of the adoption of guidelines for elective surgery in New Zealand where, as we noted earlier, the approach used was inconsistent with the experience and judgement of clinicians. In both cases, the authors point to the risks of gaming by clinicians as a way round the imposition of unacceptable guidelines.

Notwithstanding this observation, the commitment to make use of guidelines appears to be gathering momentum. This is certainly the case in New Zealand where the National Health Committee has attached particular importance to guidelines both in relation to elective surgery and more generally as a way of promoting the rational use of resources. The same applies in the United States where managed care plans seek to reduce variations in clinical practice patterns by ensuring conformity with evidence-based guidelines. Daniels draws on research into the experience of these plans to suggest how the use of guidelines to limit the provision of services can be given greater legitimacy. As he emphasizes, it is not sufficient for guidelines to remain in the professional domain. For treatment decisions based on guidelines to be seen to be fair and consistent by patients, it is important that the basis on which they have been constructed is transparent and open to challenge. In making this point, he is echoing Klein's argument that the process of decision making needs to generate socially acceptable decisions.

HEALTH TECHNOLOGY ASSESSMENT

The interest shown in guidelines is part of the wider development of evidence-based medicine and health technology assessment.

Many of the chapters in this book testify to the role of health technology assessment in rationing, at the same time highlighting its limitations. The need for medicine to be evidence-based and to draw on the results of technology assessments is underlined by Garratini and Bertele's account of the Di Bella case in Italy. In this case, the use of novel treatments for cancers and other conditions attracted extensive interest. Public demand to have access to these treatments put pressure on politicians and stimulated widespread media coverage. When the results of clinical trials became available, the limitations of the treatments were revealed but not before considerable effort and expense had been incurred.

One way of avoiding these difficulties may be to follow the example of the United States described by Clancy and Danis. This involves linking rationing decisions with the acquisition of evidence on effectiveness. The example they give is lung-volume reduction for end-stage emphysema. Initially, access to this procedure was unrestricted but it has now been agreed that Medicare patients will only have treatment reimbursed if they are enrolled in a clinical trial. By linking the funding of new technologies to a commitment to assess their effectiveness, it may be possible to ensure the managed entry of new procedures into practice. This would also address the challenge identified by Daniels of how to reassure patients with life-threatening conditions who have exhausted standard therapies that innovative treatments are being denied on cost grounds rather than on the basis of evidence.

Yet even if this were to happen, it would still not eliminate differences between clinicians on when it is appropriate to offer certain treatments. The importance of these differences is shown by the Child B case in the United Kingdom. Ham's review of this case points out that the paediatricians involved in the treatment of Child B took a different view from that of adult specialists and their counterparts in the United States on the most appropriate way of responding to the return of Child B's leukaemia. One of the reasons for this was the absence of a good evidence base in an area of treatment that was experimental. There were also differences between clinicians in estimating the likelihood that Child B would come through further intensive treatment successfully and on the balance of benefit and harm involved in attempting such treatment. In essence, in this example of rationing at the micro level, clinical judgement held the key to determining what should be done. Differences in judgement between clinicians coupled with a father prepared to use the Internet and other sources to gather his own evidence meant that the case was resolved in the public eye rather than the privacy of the consulting room.

In the case of Canada, Martin and Singer argue that approaches drawn from evidence-based medicine and cost-effectiveness analysis have been particularly influential in rationing. However, using the example of cancer care, they suggest that there is often a gap between health technology assessment carried out from a research base and decisions as they present themselves to clinicians and managers. Martin and Singer propose a closer link between different disciplinary perspectives, bringing together not only economics and clinical research but also philosophy and politics. In making this point they are reinforcing the conclusion of both Daniels and Ham that it is the combination of evidence drawn from health technology assessments and transparency about this evidence that contributes to legitimate decision making. Put another way, and to return to an earlier theme, what is important is to pay attention to both techniques and processes in the search for more effective approaches to priority setting.

ETHICS AND VALUES

The ethical dilemmas inherent in rationing emerge as a constant refrain of this book. Fundamentally, these dilemmas arise because the need to make choices on the allocation of resources almost invariably provokes debate about the principles or values that should inform these choices. In some cases, these principles or values are explicit, in others they are implicit. Either way those responsible for rationing at different levels are involved in making moral decisions, whether they recognize this or not. These decisions take many different forms including judgements about how many resources should be committed to the treatment of individual patients and how to ensure that the health of populations is maximized with the available resources. The ethical dilemmas that ensue are not new but they have assumed renewed significance in circumstances in which there is a growing gap between the demand for health care and the availability of resources.

This emerges strongly from the contribution by Williams and Yeo. These authors describe the process of regionalization in Canada which is placing responsibility for rationing on regional boards. As Williams and Yeo emphasize, ethical issues that arise for regional boards encompass both substantive questions about the goals of health care and how these should be met, and procedural issues concerning how these questions are resolved. They argue that

> In a pluralist society, it may be impossible to achieve meaning-ful consensus on many substantive issues. However, even if there is no 'right' answer, this does not mean that all answers are equally valid. Particularly in cases where consensus does not exist, decision makers should strive for 'morally defensi-ble' decisions, that is, decisions for which all relevant consider-ations have been duly entertained and the justificatory reasons have been clearly laid out (p. 126).

Griffiths and colleagues provide a practical illustration of how the equivalent of a regional board in the United Kingdom National Health Service is grappling with these issues. As they show, the use of an ethical framework in the decision-making process of the Oxfordshire Health Authority has been helpful in enabling those charged with responsibility for decision making to make morally defensible decisions. The priorities forum in Oxfordshire fulfils many of the conditions set out by Williams and Yeo for Canada and demonstrates how an ethical perspective can make a contribution in practice as well as in theory. It also shows the potential for cross-national learning.

In drawing attention to the importance of decision-making pro-cesses, these authors lend weight to the arguments of Daniels whose work, reported here and elsewhere (Daniels and Sabin 1997, 1998a), has focused particularly on this issue. Basing his obser-vations on research into rationing in managed care organizations in the United States, Daniels argues that market accountability is insufficient to ensure fairness or legitimacy of priority-setting de-cisions. Instead, he makes the case for 'accountability for reason-ableness', by which he means that decision makers have to explain the rationales for their decisions, demonstrating that these are reasonable and allowing opportunity for challenge and dispute res-olution. The frequency with which these ideas are referred to by other contributors suggests not only that the relevance of the ethi-cal dimension of priority setting is increasingly recognized but also that the arguments advanced by Daniels have purchase in a range of different systems.

One example is the United Kingdom where the Child B case reviewed by Ham indicates that accountability for reasonableness is just as important in a tax-funded national health service as it is in a privately funded fragmented health service of the kind that exists in the United States. The Child B case also illustrates an enduring ethical dilemma, namely the difficulty of weighing the needs of an individual against those of the community. In this case, the health authority responsible for making the decision at the meso level had to consider the claims of a critically ill child with a poor prognosis in the context of its duty to the population as a whole. While the rule of rescue suggested that the use of resources on this child was justified because the alternative was certain death, the health authority decided on the basis of clinical advice that further intensive treatment was not appropriate. In so doing, it was acutely aware of the opportunity costs of spending a significant sum of money on a single patient. The difficulty of achieving consensus in this case supports the observation of Williams and Yeo that decisions of this kind may often be contested in a pluralist society. As such, they also underline Klein's argument that even where information about costs and outcomes is available, the interpretation of this information, which may itself be incomplete, may be disputed.

PROCESS

To make this point is to demonstrate that discussion of the ethics of rationing and of decision-making processes are closely linked. In relation to process, Holm's claim that rationing in the Nordic countries is entering a second phase stems from the interest shown in those countries in the development of more rigorous methods for making choices. This is particularly the case in Norway where the 1997 report of the Lonning Commission

> recommends a fundamental revision of the system for setting priorities. Instead of a top-down system with one overarching definition of necessary treatment and care, a bottom-up system is recommended based on specialty-specific working groups. Each working group is given the task of explicating the specific meaning of the concepts of severity, utility, and efficiency within its specialty. From these definitions the groups should move on to suggest a ranking of the various conditions treated within the specialty, and make recommendations concerning changes in priority. These recommendations are passed on to the political level which makes the actual priority decisions . . . One of the effects of the implementation of this system would

be that both the professional groups and the politicians and administrators would have to state their reasons for making allocation decisions in a very explicit way (pp. 34–5).

Holm points out that the report of the Danish group on rationing also focused on process and he generalizes from this experience to suggest that the key characteristics of the second phase of rationing are the adoption of transparent and accountable processes.

In developing these arguments, Holm acknowledges the influence of Daniels's work in the Nordic countries. Daniels himself advances a series of specific suggestions for implementing transparent and accountable processes, namely:

1 *Publicity*: decisions regarding coverage for new technologies (and other limit-setting decisions) and their rationales must be publicly accessible.

2 *Reasonableness*: the rationales for coverage decisions should aim to provide a *reasonable* construal of how the organization should provide 'value for money' in meeting the varied health needs of a defined population under reasonable resource constraints. Specifically, a construal will be 'reasonable' if it appeals to reasons and principles that are accepted as relevant by people who are disposed to finding terms of co-operation that are mutually justifiable.

3 *Appeals*: there is a mechanism for challenge and dispute resolution regarding limit-setting decisions, including the opportunity for revising decisions in light of further evidence or arguments.

4 *Enforcement*: there is either voluntary or public regulation of the process to ensure that conditions 1–3 are met (p. 92).

Daniels emphasizes that the purpose of proposing these conditions is in part to generate legitimacy for decisions and in part 'to convert private MCO (managed care organization) solutions to problems of limit setting into part of a larger public deliberation about a major, unsolved public policy problem' (p. 94).

A number of authors link the debate about process to the issue of public involvement to suggest that explicit rationing with widespread participation offers an opportunity to inform and educate the public about the need to set limits to health care provision. Both Daniels and Sabin adopt this stance, acknowledging the challenge that exists in changing public attitudes, especially in the United States, but maintaining that only if this challenge is faced directly is there any possibility of moving the debate forward. These views are endorsed by a number of the European authors including Norheim who draws on the work of Daniels and Sabin to argue the case for transparency and accountability as a way of fostering deliberative democracy. There are echoes here of the work of Fleck (1992), who has called for an informed democratic consensus model in which through broad mechanisms of public deliberation there is debate about how limited health care resources can be distributed in a way which is both fair and cost-effective. In Fleck's view, such a model is preferable to rationing by the market, clinicians and bureaucrats.

OTHER THEMES

Two themes come out of the book that were not addressed in the Introduction. The first concerns the role of the law in rationing. This emerges strongly from the chapters on Israel, Italy and the Child B case, each of which show how patients and their families used the courts (with varying degrees of success) to challenge decisions to restrict the provision of services. It can be anticipated that legal challenges to rationing decisions will increase and this reinforces the need to ensure that the process of arriving at decisions is fair and transparent.

The second theme relates to the role of the media. Several authors comment on the manner in which the media reported examples of rationing, often in a way which did not present a balanced account of the issues. To quote Edgar:

> The role of the media is vital in having a better informed public discussion on the issues. In some cases, I believe that the New Zealand public has been badly served by the media. Health stories often focus on the exceptions. Sensational headlines frequently do not reflect the content of stories. Significantly also, the media are constrained by privacy laws from being able to report fully (p. 187).

These comments are reinforced by a detailed study of the way in which the media in the United Kingdom covered the Child B case which concluded:

> Our study suggests that while the media may raise awareness of the issues which need debating, and may influence people's perceptions of these issues they do not provide the solid base

of information which would allow people to participate in debates in a particularly informed way, and their coverage itself does not constitute a full public debate.

(Entwistle *et al.* 1996: 157)

There are important implications here for those who argue the case for democratic deliberation.

CONCLUSION

Against the background of these lessons from experience, what then are the implications for those involved in rationing and for researchers into health policy? Our assessment is that the work reported here sheds light on policy making both as an exercise in puzzling and learning and as an example of bargaining between different interests. There are as many similarities as differences between countries in the work that has been done so far, and the opportunity for ideas to be shared, and where appropriate trans-ferred, are considerable. To be sure, it is easier to describe what has been done than to evaluate success but the importance of descrip-tive accounts should not be underestimated at a time when interest in rationing is growing rapidly.

Equally, it would be wrong to take too benign a view of the policy process. It is not necessary to subscribe to a view of politics as red in tooth and claw to recognize that much of the work in this field illustrates the quest for power and influence in the health sector. Thus, there are examples of politicians challenging the influence of doctors, patients questioning the decisions of politicians and doc-tors, and the courts and the media introducing their particular forms of accountability into the process. One of the puzzles in this context is the apparent willingness of politicians to be brave (or foolish, depending on your point of view) in some systems, but not in others, by encouraging explicit rationing. The point here is that explicitness tends to enhance accountability by making transparent the location and basis of decisions and runs counter to the blame-avoidance strategies that often motivate political action (Weaver 1986).

Having made this point, there is evidence that the learning that has occurred in recent years has led to a retreat from explicitness in some countries, stimulated in part by the political costs incurred. The renewed (or in some cases continuing) focus on the micro level of rationing can be seen as an example of blame avoidance as decision makers respond to the political costs of being explicit about priorities at the macro level by shifting (or maintaining) the emphasis and responsibility to clinical decision making at the micro level. Studies of retrenchment in welfare provision (of which health service rationing are a subset) have analysed in detail the tactics available to politicians who seek to avoid unpopularity by obfuscation and other means. One of the most common tactics has been described as 'burden shifting, that is, passing responsibility for imposing cutbacks on local officials, who may then attract some of the blame' (Pierson 1994: 21). This applies as much to shifting the burden of responsibility for rationing to doctors as to local administrative agencies such as sickness funds or health authorities.

One of the effects of such an approach is to direct attention away from relatively visible and accountable decision makers to a much more diffuse group. The implication is that explicit rationing at a macro level may be difficult to sustain and that the recent interest shown in such an approach may be a temporary aberration in a much longer history of muddling through and evading responsibility. Furthermore, in those countries like the United States which (with limited exceptions such as Oregon) have chosen not to ration explicitly there remain fundamental political obstacles to adopting a different approach. As Morone has noted, 'The American way of rationing is to decentralize (in political terms hide) the choices; the result is rationing through an accumulation of narrow public policies, private decisions, and luck' (Morone 1992: 1933). This is because in the United States 'attempts to ration health care explicitly are political dynamite' (*ibid.*). In other countries where rationing is debated more openly the policy response may involve less the assumption by politicians of responsibility for decision making than the creation of agencies one step removed from government to address these issues. A recent example is the decision of the United Kingdom government to establish the National Institute for Clinical Excellence to advise on the use of resources in the National Health Service.

The introduction of agencies like the National Institute for Clinical Excellence is an example, in Klein's terms, of the concern to strengthen the institutional basis of rationing. The issue this raises is what the prospects are for using these institutions to promote democratic deliberation on rationing. The rationale for encouraging democratic deliberation is that choices in health care involve moral issues which should be neither hidden nor fudged (Fleck 1992).

What matters is to construct a process to enable deliberation to occur and to ensure participation by the public as well as experts. While there remain formidable obstacles in developing such a process, there are also risks in not doing so. Specifically, if those responsible for rationing at different levels continue to obfuscate and fail to confront the dilemmas involved directly then public confidence in the legitimacy of decisions and those charged with making them may be undermined. In this sense, the case for explicit and accountable rationing is at root an argument to maintain and in some cases restore faith in the political system.

In concluding this review of the experience reported here, we would echo the arguments of Martin and Singer who extend the analysis of Holm to suggest that what is needed in future is a third phase in the rationing debate which goes beyond the extremes of explicit/implicit, techniques/judgement and similar (artificial) dichotomies to seek a synthesis which reflects the complexities that exist in practice. Such a synthesis, we would add, should also acknowledge the twin elements of learning and bargaining which pervade this field.

REFERENCES

Aaron, H.J. (1998). Less is more: after the Clinton plan, let's think small. In S.H. Altman, U.E. Reinhardt and A.E. Shields (eds), *The Future US Health Care System: Who Will Care for the Poor and Uninsured?* Chicago, IL: Health Administration Press.

Aaron, H.J. and Schwarz, W.B. (1984). *The Painful Prescription. Rationing Hospital Care*. Washington, DC: The Brookings Institution.

Abrams, H.S. (1993). Harvard Community Health Plan's mental health redesign project: A managerial and clinical partnership. *Psychology Quarterly*, 64, 12–31.

Arnstein, S. (1969). A ladder of citizen participation in the USA. *Journal of the American Institute of Planners*, 35, 216–24.

Arrow, K.J. (1963a). *Social Choice and Individual Values*, 2nd edn. New Haven: Yale University Press.

Arrow, K.J. (1963b). Uncertainty and the welfare economics of medical care. *The American Economic Review*, 53, 941–68.

Ayanian, J. and Epstein, A. (1991). Differences in the use of procedures between men and women hospitalized for coronary artery disease. *New England Journal of Medicine*, 325(4), 221–5.

Ayanian, J.Z., Udvarhelyi, S., Gatsonis, C.A., Pahos, C.L. and Epstein, A.M. (1993). Racial differences in the use of revascularization procedures after coronary angiography. *Journal of the American Medical Association*, 269(20), 2642–6.

Bailey, M.A. (1994). The Democracy Problem. *Hastings Center Report* 24(4), 39–42.

Bankowski, Z., Bryant, J.H. and Gallagher, J. (eds) (1997). *Ethics, Equity and Health for All*. Proceedings of the 29th CIOMS Conference, Geneva.

Baron, J. (1995). Blind justice: Fairness to groups and the do-no-harm principle. *Journal of Behavioural Decision Making*, 8, 71–83.

Battista, R.N. (1996). Towards a paradigm for technology assessment. In

M. Peckham and R. Smith (eds), *Scientific Basis of Health Services*. London: BMJ Publishing Group.

Berwick, D.M. (1996). Payment by capitation and the quality of care. *New England Journal of Medicine*, 335(16), 1227–31.

Berwick, D., Hiatt, H., Janeway, P. and Smith, R. (1997). An ethical code for everybody in health care. *British Medical Journal*, 315, 1633–4.

Bin Nun, G. and Ben Ori, D. (1997). *Trends in the National Expenditure on Health*. Jerusalem: Ministry of Health.

Bland, J.M. and Altman, D.G. (1986). Statistical methods for assessing agreement between two methods of clinical measurement. *Lancet*, i, 307–10.

Blendon, R.J., Brodie, M., Benson, J.M. *et al.* (1998). Understanding the managed care backlash. *Health Affairs*, 17(4), 80–94.

Bodenheimer, T. (1997). The Oregon health plan – lessons for the nation. First of two parts. *New England Journal of Medicine*, 337, 651–5.

Bodenheimer, T. and Sullivan, K. (1998). How large employers are shaping the health care marketplace. First of two parts. *New England Journal of Medicine*, 338, 1003–7.

Boehm, T., Folkman, J., Browder, T. and O'Reilly, M.S. (1997). Antiangiogenic therapy of experimental cancer does not induce acquired drug resistance. *Nature*, 390, 404–7.

Bond, A. and Lader, M. (1974). The use of analogue scales in rating subjective feelings. *British Journal of Medical Psychology*, 47, 211–18.

Borody, J. and Gieni, K.J. (1998). Surviving change: one District Health Board's experience. *Healthcare Management Forum*, 11(2), 33–8.

Bowling, A., Jacobson, B. and Southgate, L. (1993). Explorations in consultation of the public and health professionals on priority setting in an inner London health district. *Social Science and Medicine*, 37(7), 851–7.

Brown, C.V. and Jackson, P.M. (1978). *Public Sector Economics*. Oxford: Martin Robertson.

Bryant, J., Khan, K., Marsh, D. *et al.* (1993). A developing country's university oriented toward strengthening health systems: Challenges and results. *American Journal of Public Health*, 83, 1537–43.

Calabresi, G. and Bobbitt, P. (1978). *Tragic Choices*. New York: Norton.

Campbell, A.V. (1995). Defining core health services: The New Zealand experience. *Bioethics*, 9(3/4), 252–8.

Carver, J. (1990). *Boards that Make a Difference*. San Francisco: Jossey-Bass Inc.

Casebeer, A.L. and Hannah, K.J. (1998). Managing change in the context of health reform: Lessons from Alberta. *Healthcare Management Forum*, 11(2), 21–7.

Chang, R. (ed.) (1997). *Incommensurability, Incomparability, and Practical Reason*. Cambridge, MA: Harvard University Press.

Chinitz, D. (1995). Israel's health policy breakthrough: The politics of reform and the reform of politics. *Journal of Health Policy, Politics and Law*, 20(4), 909–32.

Chinitz, D. and Israeli, A. (1997). Health reform and rationing in Israel. *Health Affairs*, 16(5), 205–10.

Chinitz, D., Shelev, C., Galai, N. and Israeli, A. (1998). Israel's basic basket of health service: The importance of being explicitly implicit. *British Medical Journal*, 317, 1005–7.

Churchill, L.R. (1987). *Rationing Health Care in America. Perceptions and Principles of Justice*. Notre Dame, IN: Notre Dame Press.

Clark, T.M. (1974). Can you cut a budget pie? *Policy and Politics*, 3(2), 3–31.

Coast, J. (1997). Rationing should be made explicit at all levels of NHS decision making: The case against. *British Medical Journal*, 314, 1118–22.

Coast, J., Donovan, J.L. and Frankel, S.J. (1996). *Priority Setting: The Health Care Debate*. Chichester: John Wiley and Sons.

Cohen, A. (1997). Promise me I will get better. *Maariv,* 10 December (Hebrew).

Collins, J.C. and Porras, J.I. (1997). *Built to Last: Successful Habits of Visionary Companies*. New York: Harper Business.

Commission on Health Research for Development (1990). *Health Research: Essential Link to Equity* in Development. New York: Oxford University Press, 43–4.

Cooper, P.F. and Schone, B.S. (1997). More offers, fewer takers for employment-based health insurance: 1987 and 1996. *Health Affairs,* 16(6), 142–9.

Copeland, C. and Pierron, B. (1998). *Implications of ERISA for Health Benefits and the Number of Self-Funded ERISA Plans,* EBRI Issue Brief. Washington, DC: Employee Benefit Research Institute.

Crawshaw, R., Garland, M.J., Hines, B. and Lobitz, C. (1985). Oregon Health Decisions: An experiment with informed community consent. *Journal of the American Medical Association,* 254, 3213–6.

Daniels, N. (1985). *Just Health Care*. New York: Cambridge University Press.

Daniels, N. (1986). Why saying no to patients in the United States is so hard: Cost containment, justice, and provider autonomy. *New England Journal of Medicine,* 314, 1381–3.

Daniels N. (1994). Four unsolved rationing problems: A challenge. *Hastings Center Report*, 24, 27–9.

Daniels, N. (1996). Justice, fair procedures, and the goals of medicine. *Hastings Center Report*, 26(6), 10–12.

Daniels, N. (1997). Limits to health care: Fair procedures, democratic deliberation and the legitimacy problem for insurers. *Philosophy and Public Affairs*, 26, 303–50.

Daniels, N., Light, D.K. and Caplan, R.L. (1996). *Benchmarks of Fairness for Health Care Reform*. New York: Oxford.

Daniels, N. and Sabin, J. (1995). The yin and yang of health care system reform. Professional and political strategies for setting limits. *Archives of Family Medicine*, 4, 67–71.

Daniels. N. and Sabin, J. (1997). Limits to health care: fair procedures, democratic deliberation, and the legitimacy problem for insurers. *Philosophy and Public Affairs*, 26(4), 303–50.

Daniels, N. and Sabin, J. (1998a). The ethics of accountability in managed care reform. *Health Affairs*, 17(5), 50–64.

Daniels, N. and Sabin, J. (1998b). Closure, fair procedures, and setting limits within managed care organizations. *Journal of the American Geriatrics Society*, 46(3), 351–4.

Daniels, N. and Sabin, J. (1998c). Last chance therapies and managed care: Pluralism, fair procedures, and legitimacy. *Hastings Center Report*, 28(2), 27–41.

Danish Council of Ethics (1996). *Priority-setting in the Health Service – A Report*. Copenhagen: Danish Council of Ethics.

Dawes, R.M. and Corrigan, B. (1974). Linear models in decision making. *Psychology Bulletin*, 81(2), 95–106.

Deber, R., Narine, L., Baranek P. *et al.* (1997). *The Public/Private Mix in Health Care*. Ottawa: National Forum on Health.

Dennett, E.R. and Parry, B.R. (1998). Generic surgical priority criteria scoring system: The clinical reality. *New Zealand Medical Journal*, 111, 163–6.

Dennett, E.R., Kipping, R.R., Parry, B.R. and Windsor, J.A. (1998). Priority access criteria for elective cholecystectomy: A comparison of three scoring methods. *New Zealand Medical Journal*, 111, 231–3.

Dixon, J. and Welch, G.H. (1991). Priority setting: Lessons from Oregon. *Lancet*, 337, 891–4.

Donaldson, C. (1995). Distributional aspects of willingness to pay. Paper presented to the Health Economists' Study Group, Aberdeen, July.

Doyal, L. (1997). Rationing within the NHS should be explicit. The case for. *British Medical Journal*, 314, 1114–18.

Draper, H. and Tunna, K. (1996). *Ethics and Values for Commissioners*. Leeds: Nuffield Institute for Health.

Drummond, M. (1998). Evidence-based medicine and cost-effectiveness: Uneasy bedfellows? *Evidence-Based Medicine*, 3(5), 133.

D'Souza, R. (1997). Household determinants of childhood mortality: illness management in Karachi Slums. PhD thesis, Australian National University, National Center for Epidemiology and Population Health, Canberra.

Dunkerley, D. and Glasner, P. (1998). Empowering the public? Citizens' juries and the new genetic technologies. *Critical Public Health*, 8(3), 181–92.

Dunning, A. (1996). Reconciling macro- and micro-concerns: Objectives and priorities in health care. In OECD, *Health Care Reform: The Will to Change*. Paris: OECD.

Eddy, D.M. (1990a). Clinical decision making: From theory to practice. Guidelines for policy statements: The explicit approach. *Journal of the American Medical Association*, 263, 2239–40, 2243.

Eddy, D.M. (1990b). Clinical decision making: From theory to practice. Practice policies – guidelines for methods. *Journal of the American Medical Association*, 263, 1839–41.

Edgar, W. (1999). Rationing health care in New Zealand – how the public has a say. Presentation at the 2nd International Conference on Priorities in Health Care, London, 8–10 October.

Elster, J. (1992). *Local Justice: How Institutions Allocated Scarce Goods and Necessary Burdens*. New York: Russell Sage Foundation.

Entwistle, V.A. *et al.* (1996a). Media coverage of the Child B case. *British Medical Journal*, 312, 1587–91.

Entwistle, V.A. *et al.* (1996b). The media and the message. In M. Marinker (ed.), *Sense and Sensibility in Health Care*. London: British Medical Journal Publishing Group.

Epstein, A.M. (1998). Rolling down the runway. The challenges ahead for quality report cards. *Journal of the American Medical Association*, 279, 1691–6.

Evans, R.G. and Wolfson, A.D. (1980). *Faith, Hope and Charity: Health Care in the Utility Function*. Vancouver: University of British Columbia.

Ezekiel, J.E. and Ezekiel, L.L. (1996). What is accountability in health care? *Annals of Internal Medicine*, 124(2), 229–39.

Feuerstein, M.T. (1980). Community participation in evaluation: Problems and potentials. *International Nursing Review*, 27(6), 187.

Fleck, L.M. (1992). Just health care rationing: A democratic decision making approach. *University of Pennsylvania Law Review*, 140(5), 1597–636.

Fleck, L.M. (1994). Just caring: Oregon, health care rationing, and informed democratic deliberation. *Journal of Medicine and Philosophy*, 19(4), 367–88.

Fleming, C., D'Agostino, R.B. and Selker, H.P. (1991). Is Coronary-Care-Unit admission restricted for elderly patients? A multicenter study. *American Journal of Public Health*, 81, 1121–6.

Forrow, L. and Side, I.V. (1998). Medicine and nuclear war, from Hiroshima to mutual assured destruction to abolition 2000. *Journal of the American Medical Association*, 280, 467.

Forrow, L. *et al.* (1998). Special report: Accidental nuclear war – a post-Cold War assessment. *New England Journal of Medicine*, 338, 1326–31.

Gold, M.R., Hurley, R., Lake, T., Ensor, T. and Berenson, R. (1995). A national survey of the arrangements managed-care plans make with physicians. *New England Journal of Medicine*, 33(25), 1678–83.

Grimes, D.S. (1987). Rationing health care. *Lancet* i, 615–16.

Grimley Evans, J. (1993). Health care rationing and elderly people. In M. Tunbridge (ed.), *Rationing of Health Care in Medicine*. London: Royal College of Physicians of London.

Gutman, A. and Thompson, D. (1996). *Democracy and Disagreement*. Cambridge, MA: Belknap Press of Harvard University Press.

Hadorn, D. (1991). Setting health care priorities in Oregon. Cost effectiveness meets the rule of rescue. *Journal of the American Medical Association*, 265, 2218–25.

Hadorn, D. (1992). Emerging parallels in the American health care and legal-judicial systems. *American Journal of Law and Medicine*, XVIII (1 and 2), 73–96.

Hadorn, D.C. and Holmes, A.C. (1997). The New Zealand priority criteria project. Part 1: Overview. *British Medical Journal*, 314, 131–8.

Ham, C. (1993). Priority setting in the NHS: Reports from six districts. *British Medical Journal*, 307(6901), 435–8.

Ham, C. (1995). Health care rationing. *British Medical Journal*, 310, 1483–4.

Ham, C. (1997). Priority setting in health care: Learning from international experience. *Health Policy*, 42, 49–66.

Ham, C. (1998a). *Setting Priorities for Health Care: Why Government Should Take the Lead*. Belfast: Northern Ireland Economic Council.

Ham, C. (1998b). Retracing the Oregon trail: The experience of rationing and the Oregon health plan. *British Medical Journal*, 316, 1965–9.

Ham, C. and Pickard, S. (1998). *Tragic Choices in Health Care: The Story of Child B*. London: King's Fund.

Haynes, R.B., Sackett, D.L., Gray, J.M.A., Cook, D.J. and Guyatt, G.H. (1996). Transferring evidence from research into practice: 1. The role of clinical care research evidence in clinical decisions. *ACP Journal Club*, Nov/Dec: A14–16.

Hayward, R.S., Wilson, M.C., Tunis, S.R., Bass, E.B. and Guyatt, G. (1995). Users' guides to the medical literature. VIII. How to use clinical practice guidelines. A. Are the recommendations valid? The Evidence-Based Medicine Working Group. *Journal of the American Medical Association*, 274(7), 570–4.

Heclo, H. (1974). *Modern Social Politics in Britain and Sweden*. New Haven: Yale University Press.

Hellinger, F.J. (1996a). The impact of financial incentives on physician behavior in managed care plans: A review of the evidence. *Medical Care Research and Review*, 53(3), 294–314.

Hellinger, F.J. (1996b). The expanding scope of state legislation. *Journal of the American Medical Association*, 276, 1065–70.

Hoinville, G. and Courtenay, G. (1979). Measuring consumer priorities. In T. O'Riordan and R.C. D'Arge (eds), *Progress in Resource Management and Environmental Planning, Vol.1*. Chichester: Wiley.

Holm, S. (1998). Goodbye to the simple solutions: The second phase of priority setting in health care. *British Medical Journal*, 317, 1000–2.

Holmes, A. and Smith, V. (1997). When to consult communities. Wellington: National Health Committee.

Hope, T., Hicks, N., Reynolds, D.J.M., Crisp, R. and Griffiths, S. (1998). Rationing and the health authority. *British Medical Journal*, 317, 1067–9.

Howson, C.P., Reddy, K.S., Ryan, T.J. and Bale, J.R. (1998). *Control of*

Cardiovascular Diseases in Developing Countries – Research, Development, and Institutional Strengthening. Washington, DC: National Academy Press.

Huber, G.P. (1974). Multi-attribute utility models: A review of field and field-like studies. *Management Science*, 20(10), 1393–1402.

Hunter, D. (1995). Rationing: the case for 'muddling through elegantly'. *British Medical Journal*, 311, 811.

Hunter, D.J. (1993). *Rationing Dilemmas in Health Care.* Research Paper No. 8. Birmingham: National Association of Health Authorities and Trusts.

Hyder, A. (1999, in press). Priority setting in health R&D: correcting the 10/90 disequilibrium. In *10/90 Disequilibrium in Health Research.* Geneva: Global Forum for Health Research.

IFNB Multiple Sclerosis Study Group (1993). Interferon beta–1b is effective in relapsing-remitting multiple sclerosis. I. Clinical results of a multicenter, randomized, double-blind, placebo-controlled trial. *Neurology*, 43, 655–61.

IFNB Multiple Sclerosis Study Group and the University of British Columbia MS/MRI Analysis Group (1995). Interferon beta–1b in the treatment of multiple sclerosis: Final outcome of the randomized controlled trial. *Neurology*, 45, 1277–85.

Iglehart, J.K. (1996). The National Committee for Quality Assurance. *New England Journal of Medicine*, 335, 995–9.

Institute of Medicine (1998). *Improving Priority Setting and Public Input at the National Institutes of Health.* Washington, DC: National Academy Press.

Israeli, A., Chinitz, D. and Galai, N. (1997). Measuring public preferences for coverage under National Health Insurance. Draft research report submitted to the Israel National Institute for Health Policy Research (Hebrew).

Jaffery, S.N. and Korejo, R. (1993). Mothers brought dead: An inquiry into causes of delay. *Social Science and Medicine*, 36, 371.

Jones, J. and Hunter, D. (1995). Consensus methods for medical and health services research. *British Medical Journal*, 311, 376–80.

Jones, L. (1993). *The Core Debator.* Wellington: National Advisory Committee on Core Health and Disability Services.

Kahn, R.L. (1993). *The MacArthur Foundation Program in Mental Health and Human Development: An Experiment in Scientific Organization.* Chicago: MacArthur Foundation.

Kaiser Family Foundation (1997). *Harvard Survey of American's View on Managed Care* (http: //www.kff.org/archive/health_policy/mcare/macaretop.html).

Kamm, F.M. (1994). To whom? *Hastings Center Report*, 24(4), 29–32.

Kao, A.C., Green, D.C., Zaslavsky, A.M., Koplan, J.P. and Cleary, P.D. (1998). The relationship between method of physician payment and patient trust. *Journal of the American Medical Association*, 280, 1708–14.

Kassirer, J.P. (1998). Managing care – should we adopt a new ethic? *New England Journal of Medicine*, 339, 397–8.

Klein, R. (1993a). Dimensions of rationing: Who should do what? *British Medical Journal*, 307, 309–11.

Klein, R. (1993b). Rationality and rationing: Diffused or concentrated decision-making? In T. Tunbridge (ed.), *Rationing of Health Care in Medicine*. London: Royal College of Physicians of London.

Klein, R. (1995). Priorities and rationing: Pragmatism or principles? *British Medical Journal*, 311(7008), 761–2.

Klein, R. (1998). Puzzling out priorities. *British Medical Journal*, 317, 959–60.

Klein, R., Day, P. and Redmayne, S. (1996). *Managing Scarcity*. Buckingham: Open University Press.

Klevit, H.D., Bates, A.C., Castanares, T. *et al.* (1991). Prioritization of health care services: A progress report by the Oregon Health Services Commission. *Archives of Internal Medicine*, 151: 912–16.

Knesset (Israel) (1997). Economics Arrangements Bill (Hebrew).

Kouri, D., Dutchak, J. and Lewis, S. (1997). *Regionalization at Age Five: Views of Saskatchewan Health Care Decision-Makers*. Saskatoon, SK: HEALNet Regional Health Planning.

Kristoffersen, M. and Piene, H. (1997). Ventelistegarantiordningen – variasjon i andel som får ventelistegaranti. *Tidsskrift for Den Norske Lægeforening*, 117, 361–5.

Lenaghan, J. (ed.) (1997). *Hard Choices in Health Care*. London: British Medical Journal Publishing Group.

Lenaghan, J., New, B. and Mitchell, E. (1996). Setting priorities: Is there a role for citizens' juries? *British Medical Journal*, 312(7064), 1591–3.

Levinsky, N.G. (1984). The doctor's master. *New England Journal of Medicine*, 311, 1573–5.

Lissak, M. (1995). Immigrants from the former Soviet Union: Integration or isolation. In Y. Kop (ed.), *Allocation of Resources to Social Services*. Jerusalem: Center for Social Policy Studies in Israel.

Lomas, J. (1997a). Devolving authority for health care in Canada's provinces: 4. Emerging issues and prospects. *Canadian Medical Association Journal*, 156, 817–23.

Lomas, J. (1997b). Reluctant rationers: Public input to health care priorities. *Journal of Health Services Research and Policy*, 2(1), 103–11.

Lomas, J. and Rachlis, M. (1996). *Moving Rocks: Block Funding in PEI as an Incentive for Cross-sectoral Reallocations among Human Services*. Working Paper 96–7. Hamilton, ON: Center for Health Economics and Policy Analysis, McMaster University.

Lown, B., Chazov, E.I., Foege, W.H., Majeed, S.U. and Reddy, R.J. (1998). Editorial. Physicians appeal to India's and Pakistan's Prime Ministers for nuclear sanity. *Journal of the American Medical Association*, 280, 467.

McKneally, M.F., Dickens, B., Meslin, E.M. and Singer, P.A. (1997).

Bioethics for clinicians: Resource allocation. *Canadian Medical Association Journal*, 157, 163–7.

McLean, I. (1987). *Public Choice*. Oxford: Blackwell.

Maynard, A. (1997). Evidence-based medicine: An incomplete method for informing treatment choices. *Lancet*, 349, 126–8.

Mechanic, D. (1995). Dilemmas in rationing health care services: The case for implicit rationing. *British Medical Journal*, 310, 1655–9.

Mechanic, D. (1997). Muddling through elegantly: Finding the proper balance in rationing. *Health Affairs*, 16(5), 83–92.

Mendelssohn, D.C., Kua, B.T. and Singer, P.A. (1995). Referral for dialysis in Ontario. *Archives of Internal Medicine*, 155, 2473–8.

Ministry of Welfare, Health and Cultural Affairs (1992). *Choices in Health Care – A Report by the Government Committee on Choices in Health Care*. Rijswijk: Ministry of Welfare, Health and Cultural Affairs.

Mooney, G. and Lange, M. (1993). Ante-natal screening: What constitutes benefit? *Social Science and Medicine*, 37(7), 873–8.

Morone, J.A. (1992). The bias of American politics: Rationing health care in a weak state. *University of Pennsylvania Law Review*, 140(5), 1923–38.

Morreim, E.H. (1995). *Balancing Act: The New Medical Ethics of Medicine's New Economics*. Washington, DC: Georgetown University Press.

Mullen, M.A., Kohut, N., Sam, M., Blendis, L. and Singer, P.A. (1996). Access to adult liver transplantation in Canada: A survey and ethical analysis. *Canadian Medical Association Journal*, 154, 337–42.

Mullen, P.M. (1983). *Delphi-type Studies in the Health Services: The Impact of the Scoring System*. Research Report 17. Birmingham: Health Services Management Centre, University of Birmingham.

Mullen, P.M. (1998a). Is it necessary to ration health care? *Public Money and Management*, 18(1), 52–8.

Mullen, P.M. (1998b). Rational rationing. *Health Services Management Research*, 11(2), 113–23.

Mullen, P.M., Murray-Sykes, K. and Kearns, W.E. (1984). Community Health Council representation on planning teams: A question of politics. *Public Health*, 98(2), 143–51.

Murray, C.J.L. and Lopez, A.D. (1997). Alternative projections of mortality and disability by cause, 1990–2020: Global burden of disease study. *Lancet*, 349, 1498–504.

National Research and Development Centre for Welfare and Health (STAKES) (1995). *From Values to Choices*. Helsinki.

New, B. (1996). The rationing agenda in the NHS. Rationing Agenda Group. *British Medical Journal*, 312(7046), 1593–601.

New, B. (ed.) (1997). *Rationing: Talk and Action in Health Care*. London: British Medical Journal Publishing Group.

Newhouse, J.P. (1992). Medical care costs: How much welfare loss? *The Journal of Economic Perspectives*, 6(3), 3–21.

New Zealand Core Services Committee (1995). Letter, 8 November.

New Zealand Herald (1997). 6 October.

NHC (1992). *The Best of Health.* Wellington, New Zealand: National Advisory Committee on Core Health and Disability Support Services.

NHC (1993a). *The Best of Health 2.* Wellington, New Zealand: National Advisory Committee on Core Health and Disability Support Services.

NHC (1993b). *Seeking Consensus.* Wellington, New Zealand: National Advisory Committee on Core Health and Disability Support Services.

NHC (1996). *Fifth Annual Report.* Wellington, New Zealand: National Advisory Committee on Core Health and Disability Support Services.

NHC (1997). *The Best of Health 3.* Wellington, New Zealand: National Advisory Committee on Health and Disability.

Nord, E., Richardson, J., Street, A., Kuhse, H. and Singer, P. (1995). Maximizing health benefits vs. egalitarianism: An Australian survey of health issues. *Social Science and Medicine*, 41, 1429–37.

Norges Offentlige Utredninger (1987). *Retningslinjer for prioritering innen norsk helsetjeneste* (Norges Offentlige Utredninger 1987: 23). Oslo: Universitetsforlaget.

Norges Offentlige Utredninger (1997). Prioritering på ny – Gjennomgang av regningslinjer for prioriteringer innen norsk helsetjeneste (Norges Offentlige Utredninger 1997: 18). Oslo: Statens Trykning.

Norheim, O.F. (1996). *Limiting access to health care: a contractualist approach to fair rationing*, Ph.D Dissertation, Institute of Medical Ethics, University of Oslo.

Norton, A. and Stephens, T. (1995). *Participation in Poverty Assessments.* Environment Paper No. 20. Washington, DC: World Bank.

Office of Technology Assessment (1982). *Strategies of Medical Technology Assessment.* Washington, DC: Government Printing Office.

Orentlicher, D. (1996). Paying physicians more to do less: Financial incentives to limit care. *University of Richmond Law Review*, 30(1), 155–97.

Pakistan Medical Research Council (1997). *National Health Survey of Pakistan, 1990–94.* Islamabad: Pakistan Medical Research Council.

Parker, R.L. *et al.* (1983). Evaluation of program utilization and cost effectiveness. In A. Kielmann *et al., Child and Maternal Health Services in Rural India. The Narangwal Experiment. Vol. 1: Integrated Nutrition and Health Care.* Baltimore: Johns Hopkins Press.

Parkin, A. (1995). Allocating health care resources in an imperfect world. *Modern Law Review*, 58, 867–78.

Pattanaik, P.K. (1997). Some paradoxes of preference aggregation. In D.C. Mueller (ed.), *Perspectives on Public Choice.* Cambridge: Cambridge University Press.

Payer, L. (1996). *Medicine and Culture.* New York: Henry Holt and Company, Inc.

Pearson, S.D., Sabin, J.E. and Emanuel, E.J. (1998). Ethical principles to guide physician compensation systems based on capitation. *New England Journal of Medicine,* 339(10), 689–93.

PEI Health and Community Services System (1997a). *PEI System*

Evaluation Project. Vol. I: A Guide to System Evaluation: Assessing the Health and Social Services System in PEI. Charlottetown, PEI: PEI Health and Community Services System (http: //www.gov.pe.ca/ health/evaluation/index.asp).

PEI Health and Community Services System (1997b). *PEI System Evaluation Project. Vol. II: Data Collection Instruments for Evaluating Health and Social Service Systems.* Charlottetown, PEI: PEI Health and Community Services System (http: //www.gov.pe.ca/health/evaluation/ index.asp).

Peled, A. (1997). Doctors Warn: cessation of drug treatments will cause patients to die. *Maariv*, 10 December (Hebrew).

Peled, A. and Greenstein, Y. (1997). The Government decides: An additional 150 million shekels for the health basket to add 15 Drugs. *Maariv,* 15 October (Hebrew).

Perez, J. (1994). Theoretical elements of comparison among ordinal discrete multicriteria methods. *Journal of Multi-criteria Decision Analysis*, 3(3), 157–76.

Pharoah, P. and Hollingworth, W. (1996). Cost effectiveness of lowering cholesterol concentration with statins in patients with and without preexisting coronary heart disease: Life table method applied to health authority population. *British Medical Journal*, 312, 1443–8.

Pierson, P. (1994). *Dismantling the Welfare State.* Cambridge: Cambridge University Press.

Pollock, A. (1992). Local voices: The bankruptcy of the democratic process. *British Medical Journal,* 305(6853), 535–6.

Power, E.J. and Eisenberg, J.M. (1998). Are we ready to use cost-effectiveness analysis in health care decision-making? A health services research challenge for clinicians, patients, health care systems, and public policy. *Medical Care*, 36(5), MS10–17.

President's Advisory Commission (1998). *Quality First: Better Health Care for All Americans.* Final report from the President's Advisory Commission on Consumer Protection and Quality in the Health care Industry. Washington, DC: Government Printing Office.

Redmayne, S., Klein, R. and Day, P. (1993). *Sharing out Resources. Purchasing and Priority Setting in the NHS.* Birmingham: NAHAT.

Reinke, W.A. (1988). *Health Planning for Effective Management.* New York: Oxford.

Richardson, A. (1997). Determining priorities for purchasers: The public response to rationing within the NHS. *Journal of Management in Medicine*, 11(4), 222–32.

Rosenbaum, S., Johnson, K., Sonosky, C., Markus, A. and DeGraw, C. (1998). The children's hour: The state children's health insurance program. *Health Affairs*, 17(1), 75-89.

Rosenfield, P.L. (1992). The potential transdisciplinary research for sustaining and extending linkages between health and social sciences. *Social Science and Medicine*, 11, 1342–57.

Roy, D.J., Williams, J.R. and Dickens, B.M. (1994). *Bioethics in Canada*. Scarborough, ON: Prentice-Hall.

Russel, L.B., Gold, M.R., Siegel, J.E., Daniels, N. and Weinstein, M.C. for the panel on cost-effectiveness in health and medicine (1996). The role of cost-effectiveness analysis in health and medicine. *Journal of the American Medical Association*, 276, 1172–7.

Ryan, M. (1996). *Using Consumer Preferences in Health Care Decision Making: The Application of Conjoint Analysis*. London: Office of Health Economics.

Sabin, J.E. (1992). 'Mind the gap': Reflections of an American health maintenance organisation doctor on the new NHS. *British Medical Journal*, 305, 514–16.

Sabin, J.E. (1994). Caring about patients and caring about money: The American Psychiatric Association code of ethics meets managed care. *Behavioural Sciences and the Law*, 12, 317–30.

Sabin, J. and Daniels, N. (1998). Making insurance coverage for new technologies reasonable and accountable. *Journal of the American Medical Association*, 279(9), 703–4.

Sackett, D.L., Richardson, W.S., Rosenberg, W. and Haynes, R.B. (1997). *Evidence-based Medicine. How to Practice and Teach EBM*. New York: Churchill Livingstone.

Sanders, D. (1998). Primary health care 21 – everybody's business. Paper presented at the WHO Alma Ata 20th Anniversary Conference, Almati, USSR, 27–8 November.

Scandinavian Simvastatin Group (1994). Randomised trial of cholesterol lowering in 4444 patients with coronary heart disease: The Scandinavian simvastatin survival study. *Lancet*, 344, 1383–9.

Shackley, P. and Ryan, M. (1995). Involving consumers in health care decision making. *Health Care Analysis*, 3(3), 196–204.

Shalev, C. (1997). *Lessons Learned – Three Years of National Health Insurance*. Jerusalem: Association for Citizens Rights (Hebrew).

Shalev, C. and Chinitz, D. (1997). In search of equity, efficiency, universality and comprehensiveness: Health reform and managed competition in Israel. *Dalhousie Law Journal*, Fall.

Sheperd, J., Cobbe, S., Ford, I. *et al.* (1995). Prevention of coronary heart disease with privastatin in men with hypercholesterolemia. *New England Journal of Medicine*, 333, 1301–7.

Singer, P.A. (1997). Resource allocation: Beyond evidence based medicine and cost-effectiveness analysis. *ACP Journal Club*, 27(3), A16–18.

Singer, P.A. and Mapa, J. (1998). Ethics of resource allocation: Dimensions for healthcare executives. *Hospital Quarterly*, 1(4), 29–31.

Smith, R. (1998). Viagra and rationing. *British Medical Journal*, 317, 760–1.

Society of Critical Care Medicine Ethics Committee (1994). Attitudes of critical care medicine professionals concerning distribution of intensive care resources. *Critical Care Medicine*, 22, 358–62.

Sosialdepartementet (1998). Forskrifter om godtgjørelse av utgifter til viktige legemidler. Fastsatt av Sosialdepartementet den 19. desember 1984. Seneste endringer 20. desember 1995.

State of Israel (1990). *Report of the Judicial State Commission of Inquiry into the Health System*. Jerusalem: Government Printing Office (Hebrew).

Steiner, C.A., Powe, N.R., Anderson, G.F. and Das, A. (1997). Technology coverage decisions by health care plans and considerations by medical directors. *Medical Care*, 35(5), 472–89.

Steingart, R.M., Packer, M., Hamm, P. and 16 other survival and ventricular enlargement investigators (1991). Sex difference in the management of coronary artery disease. *New England Journal of Medicine*, 325(4), 226–30.

Stewart, J., Kendall, E. and Coote, A. (1994). *Citizens' Juries*. London: Institute for Public Policy Research.

Strauss, A. and Corbin, J. (1990). *Basics of Qualitative Research. Grounded Theory Procedures and Techniques*. London: Sage.

Strauss, A. and Corbin, J. (1994). Grounded theory methodology: An overview. In N.K. Denzin and Y.S. Lincoln (eds), *Handbook of Qualitative Research*. Thousand Oaks: Sage Publications.

Stronks, K., Strijbis, A.-M., Wendte, J.F. and Gunning-Schepers, L.J. (1997). Who should decide? Qualitative analysis of panel data from public, patients, healthcare professionals, and insurers on priorities in health care. *British Medical Journal*, 315, 92–6.

Sunday Star Times (1997). 12 October and 2 November.

Sveriges Offentliga Utredningar (1995). *Priorities in Health Care – Ethics, Economy, Implementation*. Stockholm: Regeringskansliets Offsetcentral.

Swedish Parliamentary Priorities Commission (1995). *Priorities in Health Care: Ethics, Economy, Implementation*. Stockholm: Ministry of Health and Social Affairs.

Tengs, T.O., Adams, M.E., Pliskin, J.S., *et al.* (1995). Five hundred life-saving interventions and their cost-effectiveness. *Risk Analysis*, 15, 369–90.

Ubel, P.A., DeKay, M.L., Baron, J. and Asch, D.A. (1996). Cost-effectiveness analysis in a setting of budget constraints: Is it equitable? *New England Journal of Medicine*, 334, 1174–7.

Ubel, P.A. and Loewenstein, G. (1995). The efficacy and equity of retransplantation: An experimental survey of public attitudes. *Health Policy*, 34, 145–51.

Ubel, P.A., Loewenstein, G., Scanlon, D. and Kamlet, M. (1996). Individual utilities are inconsistent with rationing choices: A partial explanation of why Oregon's cost-effectiveness list failed. *Medical Decision Making*, 16, 108–16.

UNICEF (1996). *The State of the World's Children*. New York: UNICEF.

Weale, A. (1990). The allocation of scarce medical resources: A democrat's dilemma. In P. Byrne (ed.), *Medicine, Medical Ethics and the Value of Life*. Chichester: Wiley.

Weaver, K. (1986). The politics of blame avoidance. *Journal of Public Policy*, 6(4), 371–98.

Werner, D. (1998). Health and equity: need for a people's perspective in the quest for world health. Paper presented at the WHO Alma Ata 20th Anniversary Conference, Almaty: Kazekistan.

WHO (World Health Organization) (1996). *Investing in Health Research and Development*. Geneva: WHO.

WHO (World Health Organization) (1997). *Health for All in the Twenty-first Century*. Geneva: WHO.

Williams, J.R., Yeo, M. and Hooper, W. (1996). Ethics for regional boards. *Leadership in Health Services*, 5(4), 22–6.

Williams, S., Seed, J. and Mwau, A. (1994). *The Oxfam Gender Training Manual*. Oxford: Oxfam UK and Ireland.

Yeo, M. (1996). The ethics of public participation. In M. Stingl and D. Wilson (eds), *Efficiency Versus Equality: Health Reform in Canada*. Halifax, NS: Fernwood Publishing.

Yeo, M., Williams, J.R. and Hooper, W. (1998). Ethics and regional health boards. In L. Groarke (ed.), *The Ethics of the New Economy*. Waterloo, ON: Wilfrid Laurier University Press.

Yin, R.K. (1994). *Case Study Research: Design and Methods*. Thousand Oaks, CA: Sage Publications.

Zweibel, N.R., Cassel, C.K. and Karrison, T. (1993). Public attitudes about the use of chronological age as a criterion for allocating health care resources. *The Gerontologist*, 33, 74–80.

INDEX

MANAGING SCARCITY
PRIORITY SETTING AND RATIONING IN THE NATIONAL
HEALTH SERVICE

Rudolf Klein, Patricia Day and Sharon Redmayne

The 'rationing' of health care has become one of the most emotive
issues of the 1990s in the UK, causing much public confusion and
political controversy. This book provides a comprehensive and critical introduction to this debate. It does so by examining the processes
which determine who gets what in the way of treatment, the decision
makers involved at different levels in the NHS and the criteria used in
making such decisions. In particular it analyses the relationship
between decisions about spending priorities (taken by politicians and
managers) and decisions about rationing care for individual patients
(taken by doctors), between explicit and implicit rationing. As well as
drawing on research-based evidence about what is happening in
Britain today, *Managing Scarcity* also looks at the experience of the
NHS since 1948 and puts the case of health care in the wider context
of publicity funded services and programmes which have to allocate
limited resources according to non-market criteria.

Managing Scarcity is recommended reading for students and
researchers of health policy, as well as health professionals and policy
makers at all levels in the NHS.

Contents
*Part 1: The context – Unpicking the notion – Politics and strategies –
Principles of resource allocation – Part 2: The NHS experience – The
NHS: a history of institutionalized scarcity – Priority setting in the new
era – Lifting the veils from rationing? – Into the secret garden – Part 3:
The way ahead – Money or science to the rescue? – What can we learn
from the others? – Policy options for the future – Appendix – Refer-
ences – Index.*

176pp   0 335 19446 X (Paperback)   0 335 19447 8 (Hardback)

HEALTH CARE REFORM
LEARNING FROM INTERNATIONAL EXPERIENCE

Chris Ham (ed.)

If you want a broad introduction to international health care reform, written by some of the best health policy analysts alive today, then this is it.

Chris Heginbotham

- What policies have been adopted to reform health care in Europe and North America?
- Which policies have worked and which have failed?
- What new initiatives are emerging onto the health policy agenda?

This book provides an up-to-date review and analysis of health care reform in five countries: Germany, Sweden, the Netherlands, the United Kingdom and the United States. It reviews the experience of introducing competition into the health service as well as policies to strengthen management and change methods of paying hospitals and doctors. The experience of each country is described by experts from the countries concerned. In this lucid introduction, Chris Ham sets out the context of reform, and in the conclusion identifies the emerging lessons.

The book provides an authoritative introduction to health care reform in Europe and North America at a time of increasing political and public interest in this field. It has been designed for students of social policy and the full range of health service practitioners on courses of professional training.

Contents
The background – The United States – The United Kingdom – Sweden – The Netherlands – Germany – Lessons and conclusions – Index.

Contributors
Reinhard Busse, Chris Ham, Bradford Kirkman-Liff, Clas Rehnberg, Freidrich Wilhelm Scwartz and Wynand van de Ven.

160pp   0 335 19889 9 (Paperback)   0 335 19890 2 (Hardback)

CRITICAL CHALLENGES FOR HEALTH CARE REFORM IN EUROPE

Richard B. Saltman, Josep Figueras and Constantino Sakellarides

This volume explores the central issues driving the present process of health care reform in Europe. More than 30 scholars and policy makers from all parts of Europe draw together the available evidence from epidemiology and public health, economics, public policy, organizational behaviour and management theory as well as real world policy making experience, to lay out the options that health sector decision-makers confront. Through its cross-disciplinary, cross-national approach, the book highlights the underlying trends that now influence health policy formulation across Europe. An authoritative introduction provides a broad synthesis of present trends and strategies in European health policy.

Contents
Introduction – Part I: The context for health reform – Part II: Demand-side strategies – Part III: Supply side strategies – Part IV: On state, citizen and society – Part V: Implementing health reform – Assessing the evidence – Index.

448pp   0 335 19970 4 (Paperback)   0 335 19971 2 (Hardback)